G. Staehler S. Pomer (Eds.)

Basic and Clinical Research on Renal Cell Carcinoma

With Contributions by
A.P. Albino P.M. Alken E.P. Allhoff P. Anglard
P. Anton N.H. Bander P. Bannasch R.P. Baum
A. Belldegrun A.J.M.C. Beniers W. Boeckmann
R.L.H. Bolhuis E. Braakman H. Brauch F.M.J. Debruyne
C.L. Finstad P. Fischer G.J. Fleuren B.A. Fox P. Frost
G. Gastl M.M. Gottesman G.P. Haas H. Heinzer
R. Hohenfellner S. Hosoe E. Huland H. Huland
W.E. Hull U. Jonas A.C. Kuesel G. Kovacs M. Lerman
M. Linehan C.S. McCune S.W. Melchior S.C. Meuer
G.H. Mickisch S.C. Müller D.M. Nanus I. Pastan
W.P. Peelen L.M. Pfeffer S. Pomer J.E. Pontes
G. Riedasch W. de Riese H.K. Schackert J.A. Schalken
J.E. Scherberich C.A. Schirren V. Schirrmacher R. Schlick
G. Staehler F. Steinbach C.G. Stief M. Stöckle S. Störkel
M. Tauber R. Thiele J.W. Thüroff K. Tory J. van Dijk
J.D.H. van Eendenburg H. Völpel S.O. Warnaar S. Weier
M. Wiesel A. Yagoda B. Zbar S.Th. Zegveld H. Zerban

With 62 Figures and 33 Tables

Springer-Verlag
Berlin Heidelberg New York
London Paris Tokyo
Hong Kong Barcelona
Budapest

Prof. Dr. med. Gerd Staehler
Priv.-Doz. Dr. med. Sigmund Pomer
Abteilung Urologie und Poliklinik
Klinikum der Ruprecht-Karls-Universität
Im Neuenheimer Feld 110, W-6900 Heidelberg, FRG

ISBN-13:978-3-642-76865-1

Library of Congress Cataloging-in-Publication Data.
Basic and clinical research on renal cell carcinoma / G. Staehler, S. Pomer, (eds.); with contributions by A.P. Albino . . . [et al.].
Includes bibliographical references and index. ISBN-13:978-3-642-76865-1
e-ISBN-13:978-3-642-76863-7 DOI: 10.1007/978-3-642-76863-7
1. Kidneys—Cancer. I. Staehler, G. (Gerd) II. Pomer, S. (Sigmund) III. Albino, A.P. [DNLM: 1 Carcinoma, Renal Cell—drug therapy. 2. Carcinoma, Renal Cell—physiopathology. 3. Carcinoma, Renal Cell—therapy. 4. Kidney Neoplasms—drug therapy. 5. Kidney Neoplasms—physiopathology. 6. Kidney Neoplasms—therapy. WJ 358 B3108]
RC280.K5B26 1992 616.99'461—dc 20

Softcover reprint of the hardcover 1st edition 1992

Typesetting: Best-Set Typesetter Ltd., Hong Kong

10/3130-5 4 3 2 1 0 – Printed on acid-free paper

Preface

There are no effective standard therapies available for patients with disseminated forms of renal cell carcinoma. However, as recent developments show, new strategies for treating patients with this malignancy can be developed through the combined efforts of scientists, urologic surgeons, and medical oncologists. This is the result of our growing understanding of the molecular and cellular events connected with the malignant transformation of renal cell carcinoma.

Cytogenetic studies have identified a basis for familial renal cancer, which in some cases occurs with features of von Hippel-Lindau disease. In sporadic renal cancer, abnormalities involving chromosome 3 have also been described extensively. Tumor supressor gene absence and inactivation have been incriminated in the carcinogenesis of the heritable and sporadic forms of this neoplasm, respectively.

Renal tumors remain chemoresistent. One possible reason for the general failure of chemotherapy in patients with metastatic renal cancer is the expression of the multiple drug resistance (MDR) gene, demonstrated in the proximal tubule of the normal nephron. The MDR gene persists in kidney tumors derived from this part of the nephron. Promising strategies dealing with MDR are currently being developed.

New cytokine-based strategies for treating patients with advanced renal cell carcinoma have recently emerged. Originally, adoptive immunotherapy involving the transfer of lymphokine-activated killer cells and interleukin-2 (IL-2) was developed. Numerous methods of cytokine administration in patients with metastatic renal cancer followed, including therapies using low IL-2 doses and topical application, both of which are associated with reduced toxicity. Randomized trials now being conducted are also expected to show improved response rates of these new treatment modalities.

Hopefully, these advances will lead to more effective treatments for renal cell carcinoma.

Heidelberg, February 1992 *G. Staehler* *S. Pomer*

Contents

Chemotherapy of Renal Cell Carcinoma

Immunobiology of Renal Cell Carcinoma

List of Contributors*

Albino A. P. 115[1]
Alken, P. M. 79
Allhoff, E. P. 61
Anglard, P. 27
Anton, P. 61
Bander, N. H. 115
Bannasch, P. 9
Baum, R. P. 148
Belldegrun, A. 200
Beniers, A. J. M. C. 121
Boeckmann, W. 148
Bolhuis, R. L. H. 156
Braakman, E. 156
Brauch, H. 27
Debruyne, F. M. J. 121
Finstad, C. L. 115
Fischer, P. 148
Fleuren, G. J. 156
Fox, B. A. 165
Frost, P. 134, 142
Gastl, G. 115
Gottesman, M. M. 89
Haas, G. P. 200
Heinzer, H. 221
Hohenfellner, R. 49
Hosoe, S. 27
Huland, E. 221
Huland, H. 221
Hull, W. E. 37
Jonas, U. 61
Kuesel, A. C. 37
Kovacs, G. 3
Lerman, M. 27
Linehan, M. 27
McCune, C. S. 189
Melchior, S. W. 49
Meuer, S. C. 101
Mickisch, G. H. 79, 89
Müller, S. C. 49
Nanus, D. M. 115
Pastan, I. 89
Peelen, W. P. 121
Pfeffer, L. M. 115
Pomer, S. 37, 212

* Addresses are given at the beginning of the respective contribution
[1] Page on which contribution begins

Molecular and Cellular Basis of Renal Cell Carcinoma

Molecular Differential Pathology of Renal Cell Tumors*

G. Kovacs[1]

There is growing evidence that alterations at specific chromosomal regions are crucial events in the initiation and progression of human cancer. Site-specific, chromosomal rearrangements involving proto-oncogenes are particularly evident in hematological malignancies. They have a strong impact on the diagnosis and classification of malignant lymphomas and leukemias.

Comprehensive cytogenetic and molecular genetic data on carcinomas and sarcomas are not yet available. At present, colon carcinoma is the most extensively characterized human solid tumor in terms of molecular genetic alterations. The familial predisposition to cancer and the opportunity to observe the stepwise genetic alteration during the transformation of normal epithelium into benign hyperplasia or adenoma and finally into a malignant carcinoma made this type of tumor attractive for molecular studies. The accumulation of genetic changes, such as mutational activation of the Ki-*ras* oncogene, loss of genetic information at chromosomal region 5q22 (the locus of familial adenomatous polyposis gene), at 17p13 (the locus of the p53 gene), and at 18q21 (*DCC* gene, i.e. deleted in color cancer), marks the development and progression of colon cancer [1].

* This project has been funded at least in part with Federal funds from the Department of Health and Human Services under contract number NO1-CO-74102 with Program Resources, Inc./DynCorp and by a grant of the German Research Council. The content of this publication does not necessarily reflect the views or policies of the Department of Health and Human Services, nor does mention of trade names, commercial products, or organizations imply endorsement by the U.S. Government.

[1] Biological Carcinogenesis and Development Program, Program Resources, Inc./DynCorp, NCI-FCRDC, P.O. Box B, Bldg. 560, Rm. 31–76, Frederick, MD 21702-1201, USA

G. Staehler S. Pomer (Eds.)
Basic and Clinical Research on Renal Cell Carcinoma

I show that molecular cytogenetics gives not only insight into events triggering the development and progression of solid tumors, but that it can be applied to the classification of neoplasms. Our combined histologic, cytogenetic, and molecular genetic analysis resulted in the identification of subtypes among renal cell tumors with distinct molecular pathology [3].

Renal Cell Tumors with Deletion of Chromosome 3p – Nonpapillary, Clear Cell Renal Cell Carcinomas (RCC)

These tumors are composed of solid, trabecular, tubular, or cystic growth of clear cells. Occasionally, some areas with tubulopapillary or papillary growth patterns may be observed. Clear cell RCCs have strong tendencies to become a diffuse or central fibrosis. They occur in either hereditary, or sporadic forms.

Hereditary, nonpapillary RCCs. The susceptibility to the development of nonpapillary RCCs might be inherited. In two families, each member carrying a germ line chromosomal mutation in the form of a balanced translocation 3;8 or 3;6 developed multiple bilateral RCCs. An autosomally inherited disorder, von Hippel-Lindau (VHL) disease, is generally manifested between the ages of 20 and 40, affecting multiple organs. The renal cysts occurring in more than 50% of VHL patients are precursor lesions for tumors, and multiple, bilateral RCCs develop in about 25%–30% of the carriers.

Sporadic nonpapillary RCCs. The vast majority of renal cell tumors with the loss of chromosome 3p segment occurs in a sporadic form. Detailed histological analyses of the entire kidney fail to detect any precursor lesions.

Genetic Changes in Nonpapillary, Clear Cell RCCs

Loss of the smallest overlapping chromosomal region of 3p13-pter occurs in over 90% of nonpapillary, clear cell RCCs [5, 7]. We have found this aberration in 81 of 85 sporadic tumors, in 8 of 8 familial RCCs, and in 40 of 40 RCCs which developed in patients with VHL disease. These data suggest that the loss of chromosome 3p segment is the highly specific chromosomal change in hereditary as well as in sporadic RCCs. Additionally, a partial trisomy of the chromosome

5q22-qter segment has been found in about 50% of the cases. The genetic mechanism resulting in the net loss of 3p and the gain of 5q segments is a mitotic chromatid exchange between the two chromosomes [4]. The most common karyotype alteration, associated with the progression of nonpapillary RCCs, is the loss of one chromosome 14. Restriction fragment length polymorphism (RELP) analysis of tumors with DNA probes mapped to the chromosomal regions in question confirms the cytogenetic findings.

Renal Cell Tumors with Trisomy 7, 17, and Loss of the Y Chromosome – Papillary Renal Cell Tumors

Papillary renal cell tumors (RCT) consist of papillary or tubulopapillary growths of small, cuboidal "basophilic" cells or large, columnar "eosinophilic" or "basophilic" cells. Compression of such structures resembles trabecular or solid patterns, and clear cell areales occasionally occur. Papillary RCTs frequently have an intratumoral lymphocytic infiltration and show a tendency to necrosis, which results in cystic changes. The development of papillary RCTs is highly associated with the presence of multiple, small precursor lesions in the same kidney. Papillary RCT develops preferentially in males; the male to female ratio is 5:1.

Genetic Changes in Papillary RCTs

Papillary RCTs are characterized by chromosomal changes distinct from those found in nonpapillary RCCS. None of the papillary RCTs shows the rearrangement of the chromosome 3p segment or the trisomy of 5q segment. These data have been confirmed by RFLP analysis using the same DNA markers which have been utilized in the study of nonpapillary RCCS. However, a trisomy 7 and 17, loss of the Y chromosome, as well as trisomy 16, 20, and 12, are specifically associated with the papillary RCTs [2].

A group of papillary RCTs is marked by a combined trisomy 7 and 17 and a loss of the Y chromosome. No other karyotype changes have been detected in these cases. The size of such tumors varies between 2 mm and 5.5 cm. Each tumor of this group shows a cytological grade G1. RFLP analysis of multiple tumors detected the duplication of the same alleles at chromosomes 7 and 17. I suggest that these tumors are benign *papillary renal cell adenomas* (RCA), irrespective of their size.

Table 1. Differential genetics of renal cell tumors

Types of tumors	Genetic alterations						
	+7	+17	−Y	+16	del(3p)	+5q	mtDNA aberration
Papillary RCTs – RCA	100%	100%	80%	–	–	–	–
– RCC	70%	80%	85%	70%	–	–	–
Nonpapillary, clear cell RCC	20%	–	25%	6%	96%	50%	–
Renal oncocytoma	–	–	–	–	–	–	100%

Another group of papillary RCTs shows genetic changes in addition to those found in tumors of the first group. The most frequent additional karyotype aberration is the trisomy of chromosome 16. Trisomy 12 or 20 might occur in combination with trisomy 16. Most tumors of this group show a cytological grade 2 or 3 and produce metastatic growth. I suggest that these tumors represent malignant *papillary RCCs*, irrespective of their size.

Renal Oncocytoma

Renal oncocytoma is a benign tumor consisting of sheets of large cells with abundant eosinophilic, granular cytoplasm. Electron microscopic analysis reveals cells that have compactly packed mitochondria with an abnormal morphology. Oncocytomas consist of a mixed cell population with normal and abnormal karyotypes. No recurrent chromosome aberration has been found. Oncocytomas have an altered restriction pattern of the mitochondrial DNA [6].

Conclusion

Recent molecular cytogenetic studies showed an impact on the classification of renal cell tumors. These findings open a new route for further molecular studies as well as for individual therapy of renal cell tumors.

Addendum. Chromophobe RCC has been identified as an entity by morphological methods. Preliminary cytogenetic, RFLP, and mitochondrial DNA analyses suggest that chromophobe RCC is an entity, characterized by an alteration of the mitochondrial as well as the chromosomal DNA (G. Kovacs, unpublished).

References

1. Fearon ER, Vogelstein B (1990) A genetic model for colorectal tumorigenesis. Cell 61: 759–767
2. Kovacs G (1989) Papillary renal cell carcinoma: A morphologic and cytogenetic study of 11 cases. Am J Pathol 134: 27–34
3. Kovacs G (1990) Application of molecular cytogenetic techniques to the evaluation of renal parenchymal tumors. Guest editorial. J Cancer Res Clin Oncol 116: 381–323

4. Kovacs G, Kung H (1991) Non-homologous chromatid exchange in hereditary and sporadic renal cell carcinomas. Proc Natl Acad Sci USA 88: 194–198
5. Kovacs G, Erlandsson R, Boldog F, Ingvarsson S, Muller-Brechlin R, Klein G, Sumegi J (1988) Consistent chromosome 3p deletion and loss of heterozygosity in renal cell carcinoma. Proc Natl Acad Sci USA 85: 1571–1575
6. Kovacs G, Welter K, Wilkens L, Blin N, DeRiese W (1989) Renal oncocytoma. A phenotypic and genotypic entity of renal parenchymal tumors. Am J Pathol 134: 967–971
7. Zbar B, Braunch H, Talmadge C, Linehan M (1987) Loss of alleles of loci on the short arm of the chromosome 3 in renal cell carcinoma. Nature 327: 721–724

Pathobiology of Renal Carcinogenesis

P. Bannasch[1] and H. Zerban

Introduction

The long-standing controversy concerning the histogenesis of kidney cancer, especially the so-called hypernephroma (which was taken for a dysontogenetic tumor by Grawitz in 1883), appeared to be settled 30 years ago when Oberling and colleagues (1960) provided persuasive evidence for an origin of the hypernephroid carcinoma from the epithelium of the proximal nephron. Consequently, the term hypernephroma was replaced by renal cell carcinoma (WHO 1981). Some findings in rodents treated with chemical carcinogens seemed for a long time to support the conception of a pivotal role of the proximal nephron in the histogenesis of renal cell tumors (Lipsky and Trump 1988). However, during the past decade, several original observations in animal models (Bannasch and Zerban 1990) and a number of new findings in man (Thoenes et al. 1986; Eble 1990; Kovacs 1990) have reopened the discussion on the cellular origin, the mechanism of development, the classification, and the prognosis of renal cell tumors.

The results of cytogenetic and molecular genetic studies suggested to some authors that specific chromosomal aberrations, especially a deletion in the short arm of chromosome 3, might play a crucial role in renal carcinogenesis and permit a subclassification in two types of renal cell carcinoma, namely nonpapillary carcinomas with and papillary carcinomas without this chromosomal change (Kovacs 1990). However, the significance of these observations is controversial since variable frequencies of the 3p deletion and other chromosomal aberrations were found in renal cell carcinomas by different groups

[1] Deutsches Krebsforschungszentrum, Abteilung für Cytopathologie, Im Neuenheimer Feld 280, W-6900 Heidelberg 1, FRG

G. Staehler S. Pomer (Eds.)
Basic and Clinical Research on Renal Cell Carcinoma

(Berger et al. 1986; Teyssier et al. 1986; Yoshida et al. 1986; Carrol et al. 1986; De Jong et al. 1988; Kovacs and Frisch 1989; Kovacs et al. 1989b; Krech et al. 1989). Krech and colleagues (1989) reported only recently that they were unable to detect any specific chromosomal aberration in renal cell carcinomas. Only 25% of the renal cell carcinomas in the material of these authors showed a rearrangement of the critical 3p segment, and there was no consistent cytogenetic difference between papillary and nonpapillary carcinomas. It is, thus, by no means obsolete to look for other cellular and subcellular criteria in order to classify renal cell tumors and to clarify their pathogenesis and prognosis.

Animal Models of Renal Carcinogenesis

In laboratory animals, particularly small rodents, the kidney has been shown to be a frequent target oı more than a hundred renotropic chemical carcinogens, different types of radiation, and some viruses (Hiasa and Ito 1987; Lipsky and Trump 1988; Bannasch and Zerban 1990). Our own experience in experimental renal carcinogenesis is based on several series of rats which were treated orally with different nitrosamines (*N*-nitrosodiethylamine, *N*-nitrosodiethanolamine, *N*-nitrosoethylethanolamine, and especially *N*-nitrosomorpholine, NNM), or received a single subcutaneous injection of 65 mg/kg streptozotocin (Bannasch et al. 1974; 1978a and b, 1979, 1980, 1988;

Table 1. Rat renal cell tumors: combined cytological and histological classification. (From Bannasch et al. 1974)

Cytology	Histology				
	Tubular/ trabecular	Solid	Cystic	Cystic-papillary	Alveolar
Clear/acidophilic (granular)	−	+	+	+	−
Acidophilic	+	+	+	+	+
Basophilic	+	+	+	+	−
Chromophobic	−	+	−	−	−
Oncocytic	−	+	+	−	−

+, positive correlation; −, negative correlation

Tsuda et al. 1986; Nogueira and Bannasch 1988; Mayer et al. 1989; Nogueira et al. 1989). Using the NNM stop model (in which the carcinogen is administered for a limited time period, 3–7 weeks, and tumor development is studied up to 2 years after withdrawal) we were able to produce in rats nearly all types of renal cell tumors (Table 1) known from human pathology including papillary and non-papillary histological variants (Bannasch and Zerban 1986; Bannasch et al. 1986b). The tumors developed only some weeks or even months after withdrawal of the carcinogen. During exposure to the carcinogen there were usually neither unspecific toxic kidney lesions, such as necrotic changes, nor proliferative tubular alterations.

However, some weeks after cessation of treatment, characteristic tumor prestages emerged which originated from specific segments of the renal tubular system (Fig. 1), indicating that differentiation of the target cells of the carcinogen plays an important role in their commitment to certain types of tumor cells. In addition to the proximal nephron, the collecting duct system was a preferred site of origin of renal cell tumors (Bannasch et al. 1989). According to cytological criteria at least four different types of preneoplastic and neoplastic renal cell lesions may be distinguished, namely, chromophobic, basophilic, clear cell/acidophilic, and oncocytic, all of which may occur concomitantly in the same kidney or bilaterally (Bannasch et al. 1974).

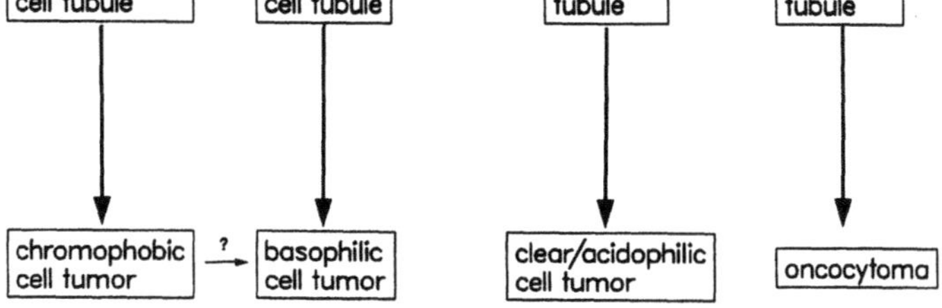

Fig. 1. Sites of origin and developmental stages of different types of rat renal cell tumors. (From Bannasch and Zerban 1990)

Chromophobic and Basophilic Cell Tubules and Tumors

In the rat, the chromophobic and the basophilic lesions derive from the proximal nephron (Fig. 1). Chromophobic cell tubules and tumors were observed after treatment of rats with NNM (Bannasch et al. 1974, 1979, 1980) and *N*-nitrosodiethylamine (Nogueira 1987). The chromophobic tubular segments consist of unusually large, polyhedral cells which sometimes show an apical brush border like normal cells of the proximal tubule (Fig. 2a). The finely reticular cytoplasm of the chromophobic cells is always PAS negative but frequently rich in substances which give a positive iron binding reaction according to Hale's iron stain or stain with alcian blue. These histochemical reactions suggest an excessive storage of mucopolysaccharides (glycosaminoglycans, proteoglycans) which are probably enclosed in cytoplasmic vacuoles as seen at the ultrastructural level. However, the histochemical reactions are not always positive. This may be due either to insufficient preservation of readily soluble polysaccharides

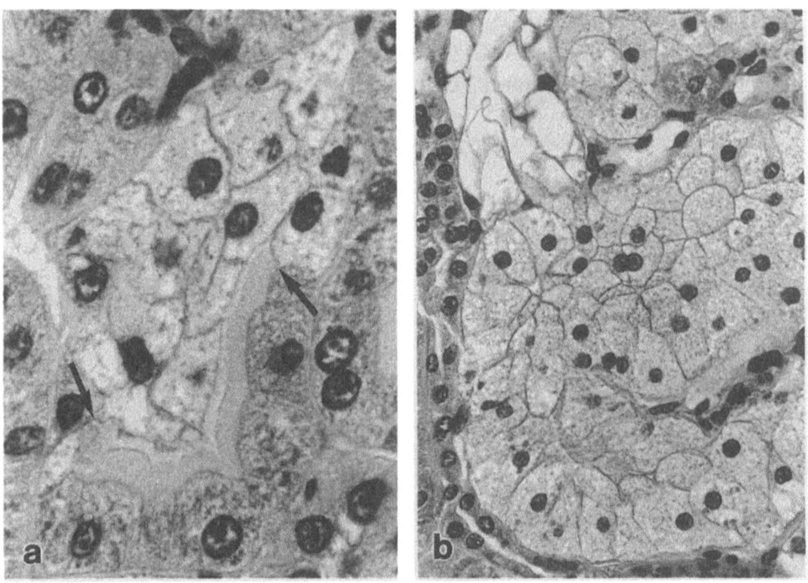

Fig. 2a, b. Chromophobic cell lesions induced in rats with *N*-nitrosomorpholine. **a** Chromophobic cells in proximal tubule. Note transition (↓) from cells of normal appearance bearing a typical brush border to chromophobic cells with a finely reticular cytoplasm and prominent nuclei. H&E, ×1100. **b** Portion of chromophobic cell tumor. H&E, ×450 or to the storage of other substances, such as lipids which are eluted during tissue preparation.

The chromophobic tubules give rise to chromophobic cell tumors (Fig. 2b) which may also store glycosaminoglycans. In the rat, the chromophobic tumors usually remain very small and can only be detected microscopically.

On the basis of our experimental findings, Thoenes and colleagues have defined and described in detail a chromophobic renal cell carcinoma as a new pathomorphologic entity in man (Thoenes et al. 1985, 1988). Although the human chromophobic tumors show many similarities to those of the rat, Störkel and coworkers (1988b) reported that they apparently do not derive from the proximal nephron but from the collecting duct system.

In rat kidney treated with various chemical carcinogens, the basophilic renal cell tumors predominate. There is circumstantial evidence that the chromophobic tubules may transform into basophilic tubules and tumors (Bannasch et al. 1980). We draw this conclusion from the frequent appearance of intermediate stages between Hale-positive and basophilic tubules and the intimate topographical association of many chromophobic tubules with basophilic tumors. However, basophilic tubules (Fig. 3a) storing low amounts of glycosaminoglycans may also derive from proximal tubules without a chromophobic intermediate stage. Transitions between such basophilic tubules and basophilic renal cell tumors have been documented by many authors (for literature see Hard 1986; Bannasch and Zerban 1990).

The definitive basophilic cell tumors (Fig. 3b) are always poor in, or free from, histochemically demonstrable mucopolysaccharides but rich in free or membrane-bound ribosomes. The presence of a prominent brush border and the frequent occurrence of peroxisomes indicate the origin of the basophilic cell tumors from the proximal nephron even at this late stage of tumor development (Bannasch et al. 1980). Similar electron microscopical observations have been reported for basophilic epithelial tumors induced in rat kidney with various other chemicals (Mao and Molnar 1967; Hard and Butler 1971a, b; McGiven and Ireton 1972; Hruban et al. 1973; Merkow et al. 1973; Gusek 1975; Dees et al. 1976).

We investigated basophilic tubules and tumors produced in rat kidney with nitrosamines (Tsuda et al. 1986) or streptozotocin (Bannasch et al. 1988; Beck 1988) by enzyme histochemical methods. Both the tubular lesions and the tumors were consistently characterized by the same enzyme-histochemical pattern (Fig. 4a–f). The activities of glucose-6-phosphatase, succinate dehydrogenase, γ-glutamyl-

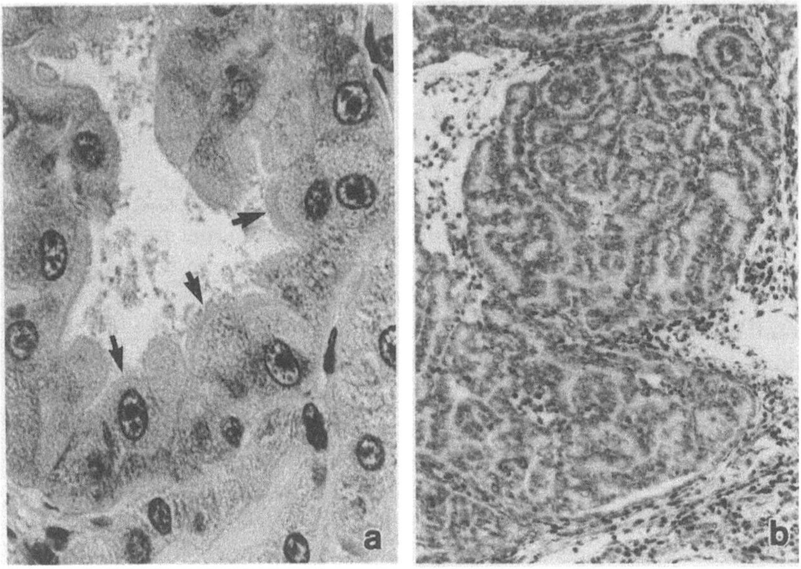

Fig. 3a, b. Basophilic cell lesions induced in rats with *N*-nitrosomorpholine. **a** Portion of basophilic cell tubule exhibiting an apical brush border (↓) and prominent nuclei. H&E, ×770. **b** Portion of basophilic cell tumor. H&E, ×170

transferase, alkaline and acid phosphatase were decreased, while those of the glyceraldehyde-3-phosphate dehydrogenase and glucose-6-phosphate dehydrogenase were increased (Table 2). These observations support the postulated histogenetic connection between basophilic tubules and tumors. They are also in line with histochemical findings in basophilic renal cell tumors induced by other chemical carcinogens (Ito et al. 1966; Mao and Molnar 1967; Jasmin and Riopelle 1969; Heatfield et al. 1976). The results of the histochemical studies suggest that a marked shift in energy metabolism from oxidative to glycolytic production of ATP, with a corresponding reduction in mitochondrial respiration, is characteristic of this tumor type. Since the pentose phosphate shunt, in addition to its other functions, provides pentoses for RNA and DNA synthesis, activation of this pathway is probably closely related both to the increase in ribosomes (basophilia) and to the enhanced cell proliferation in the basophilic lesions. A remarkable observation in the streptozotocin-induced, predominantly basophilic renal epitheliomas was the additional appearance of some clear cells storing glycogen in excess (Fig. 4b) and a strong activity of glycogen phosphorylase throughout the tumor tissue

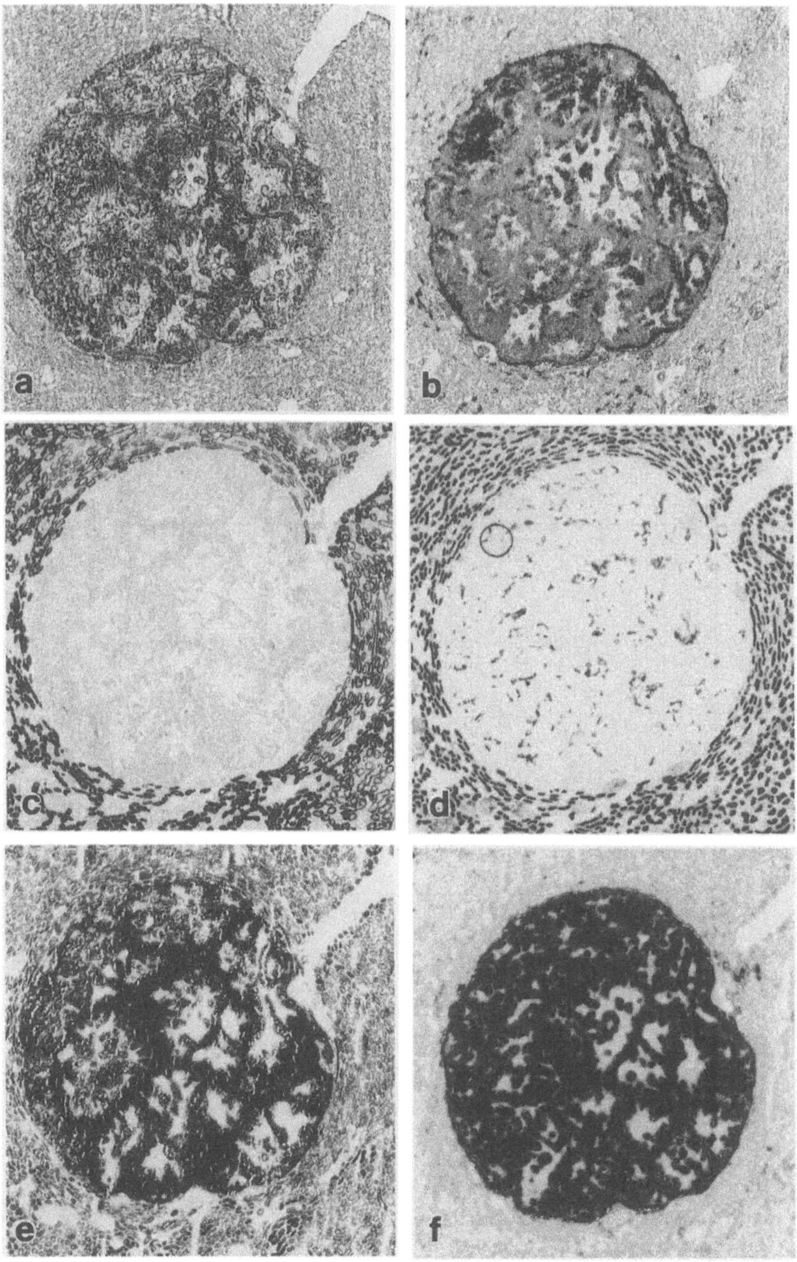

Fig. 4a–f. Histochemical pattern of basophilic cell tumor induced in rat with streptozotocin (**a–f**, serial sections). **a** Demonstration of basophilia by toluidine blue. **b** Storage of some glycogen (black) as demonstrated by the PAS reaction. **c** Decreased activity of glucose-6-phosphatase. **d** Decreased activity of adenosinetriphosphatase. **e** Increased activity of glyceraldehyde-3-phosphate dehydrogenase. **f** Increased activity of glucose-6-phosphate dehydrogenase. All figures: ×18. (From Beck 1988)

Table 2. Histochemical pattern of 20 streptozotocin-induced rat renal basophilic cell tumors as compared to that of the proximal tubule. (From Beck 1988)

	G6Pase	Syn	PHO	Gly	G6PDH	GAPDH	AC	GGT	ATPase	AlkPase	APase
1	↓	n.e.	=	=	↑	↑	↓	↓	↑	↓	↓
2	↓	=	↑	↑	↑	↑	↓	↓	↑	↓	↓ ↑
3	↓	n.e.	n.e.	↑	↑	↑	↓	↓	n.e.	↓	↓
4	↓	↑	↑	↑	↑	↑	↓	↓	↑	↓	↓ ↑
5	↓	n.e.	↑	↑	↑	↑	↓	↓	=	↓	↓ =
6	↓	↑	↑	↑	↑	↑	↓	↓	↑	↓	↓ =
7	↓	↑	↑	↑	↑	↑	↓	↓	↑	↓	↓ ↑
8	↓	↑	n.e.	↑	↑	↑	↓	↓	↑	↓	↓ ↑
9	↓	↑	↑	↑	↑	↑	↓	↓	↑	↓	↓
10	↓	↑	↑ =	↑	↑	↑	↓	↓ =	↑	↓	↑ =
11	↓	↑ =	↑ =	↑	↑	↑	↓	↓	↑	↓	↓
12	↓	↑ =	=	↑	↑	↑	↓	↓	↑ =	↓	↓
13	↓	↑ =	↑	↑	↑	↑	↓	↓	↑ =	↓	↓ =
14	↓	↑	↑	↑	↑	↑	↓	↓	↑	↓	↓
15	↓ =	=	↑ =	↑	↑	↑	↓	↓	↑	↓	↓
16	↓	↑	↑	↑	↑	↑	↓	↓	↑	↓	↓
17	↓	↑ =	↑	↑	↑	↑	↓	↓	↑ =	↓	↓
18	↓	↑ =	↑	↑	↑	↑	↓	↓	↑	↓	↓
19	↓	↑ =	↑	↑	↑	↑	↓	↓	↑	↓	↓ =
20	↓	=	↑	↑	↑	↑	↓	↓ =	↑	↓	↓ =

Enzyme activity: ↑ increased; ↓ decreased; = unchanged; n.e. not evaluable;
G6Pase, glucose-6-phosphatase; *Syn*, glycogen synthase; *PHO*, glycogen phosphorylase; *Gly*, glycogen; *G6PDH*, glucose-6-phosphate dehydrogenase; *GAPDH*, glyceraldehyde-3-phosphate dehydrogenase; *AC*, adenylate cyclase; *GGT*, γ-glutamyltransferase; *ATPase*, adenosine triphosphatase; *AlkPase*, alkaline phosphatase; *APase*, acid phosphatase

(Bannasch et al. 1988). This unusual metabolic pattern of basophilic renal cell tumors may be due to the high levels of blood glucose in these animals which suffer from streptozotocin-induced diabetes.

Clear Cell (Glycogenotic) Tubules and Clear/Acidophilic Cell Tumors

The clear and acidophilic (granular) cell tumors correspond to the predominant human renal cell carcinoma which has been known to store large amounts of glycogen and lipids for a long time. In the rat, the development of the clear and acidophilic cell tumors had been traced to clear cell tubules (Fig. 5a) which are likewise characterized by an excessive storage of glycogen (Bannasch et al. 1978a). As demonstrated in systematic studies on serial sections of more than 40 clear

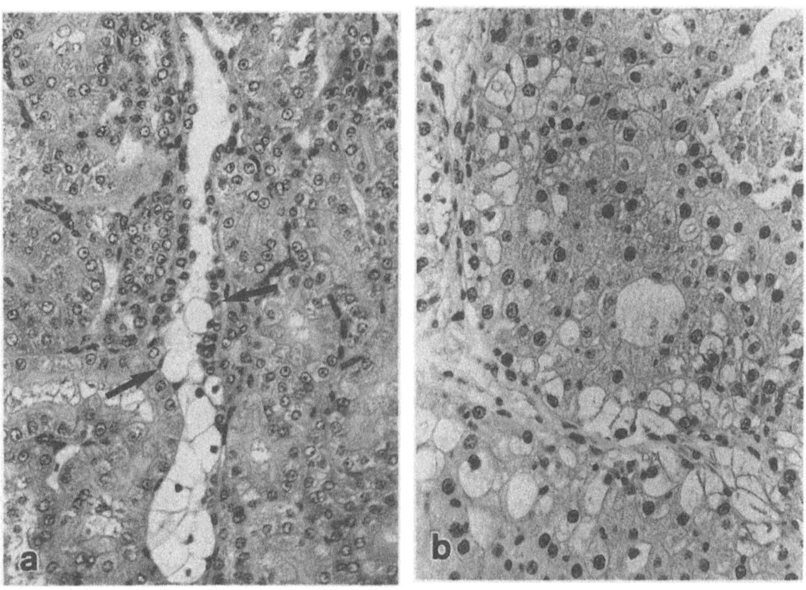

Fig. 5a, b. Clear cells in preneoplastic and neoplastic lesions induced in rat with *N*-nitrosomorpholine. **a** Cortical collecting duct partly lined by large clear cells with small condensed nuclei. Note transition (↓) from clear cells to cells of normal appearance. H&E, ×260. **b** Portion of clear/acidophilic cell tumor. Note decondensed nuclei of many acidophilic cells as compared to condensed nuclei of clear cells. H&E, ×420 cell or clear/acidophilic renal cell lesions in NNM-treated rats, all of these lesions were directly connected with the collecting duct system, especially the cortical collecting duct, but not with any other part of the tubular system (Nogueira et al. 1989). There is, thus, compelling evidence for an origin of rat renal clear cell tumors from the collecting duct system under our experimental conditions. Since this finding is at variance with the generally accepted concept that clear cell carcinomas in man derive from the proximal nephron, it should stimulate further comparative studies.

In the animal model, all intermediate stages leading from the tubules storing glycogen in excess to large tumors composed of both clear glycogen storage cells and acidophilic cells poor in glycogen but frequently exhibiting marked nuclear atypia may be observed (Fig. 5b; Bannasch et al. 1978a). There is usually a relative increase in the number of acidophilic cells with increasing tumor size. Whereas abundant glycogen and lipid bodies are found in the cytoplasm of the clear cells at the electron microscopic level, the acidophilic cells are frequently crowded with mitochondria which are characterized by a marked reduction in cristal membranes. The lipid bodies show a regular pattern of dark and light lines with a periodicity of 5–7 nm; they most probably represent glycolipids. Recently, similar osmiophilic bodies have been described in human clear cell carcinomas (Hull and Eble 1987), but this finding should not detract from the fact that the human tumors usually contain homogeneous osmiophilic droplets composed of neutral lipids.

The metabolic pattern of the rat renal clear cell and acidophilic cell tumors has not been studied in detail up to now. However, enzyme histochemical investigations in human clear cell and chromophobic cell carcinomas revealed metabolic aberrations (Table 3) similar to those presented for the basophilic renal cell tumors of the rat (Bannasch et al. 1986a). This holds particularly true for a decreased activity of the glucose-6-phosphatase and increased activity of glyceraldehyde-3-phosphate dehydrogenase, indicating a high glycolysis at the expense of gluconeogenesis. The histochemical results largely agree with biochemical data reported by Weber (1980) and obtained in our laboratory by Mayer (Mayer and Bannasch 1988), who also provided circumstantial evidence for an increased level of glucose-6-phosphate in renal cell carcinomas. Further biochemical studies are needed to find out whether changes in this central metabolite of the carbohydrate metabolism are essential in the development of the metabolic aberrations characterizing clear cell carcinomas.

Table 3. Enzyme histochemical pattern of human renal cell carcinomas. (From Bannasch et al. 1986a)

Patient no.	Age	Sex	Cell type of renal carcinoma	Evaluation of enzyme activity G6Pase	Syn	PHO	G6PDH	GAPDH	APase	GGT
1	66	♂	Clear/granular	↓↓	↑↑	↑↑	=	↑	↓	↓
2	40	♂	Granular/clear	↓↓	↑	↑	↑↑	=	↓	↓
3	53	♂	Granular	↓↓	↑↑	↑↑	=	↑	↓	↓
4	70	♂	Clear	↓↓	↑↑	↑↑	↓	↑	↓	↓
5	77	♂	Clear/granular	↓↓	↑	↑	↓	↑↑	↓	↓
6	62	♂	Clear	↓↓	↑↑	↑↑	↑	↑	↓	↓
7	83	♂	Clear	↓↓	↑↑	↑↑	=	↑	↓	↓
8	67	♂	Clear	↓↓	↑↑	↑↑	=	↑	↓	↓
9	62	♂	Clear	↓↓	↑↑	↑↑	=	↑	↓	↓
10	56	♂	Granular/clear	↓↓	↑	↑	↑	=	↓	↓
11	81	♂	Clear/granular	↓↓	↑↑	↑↑	=	↑	↓	↓
12	80	♂	Granular/clear	↓↓	↑↑	↑↑	↑↑	↑	=	↓↓
13	49	♂	Clear/granular	↓	↑↑	↑↑	↓	↑	↓	↓
14	44	♀	Clear	↓↓	↑↑	↑↑	↓	↑	↓	↓
15	52	♂	Clear/granular	↓↓	↑↑	↑↑	↑	↑↑	↓	↓
16	47	♀	Chromophobic	=	↑	↓	↑↑	↑↑	↓	↓
17	55	♂	Clear	↓↓	↑↑	↑↑	↑	↑↑	=	↓
18	53	♂	Clear	↓↓	↑↑	↑↑	↓	↑	↓	↓
19	60	♂	Clear	↓↓	↑↑	↑↑	↓	↑	↓	↓
20	78	♀	Clear	↓↓	↑↑	↑↑	↓	↑	↓	↓
21	60	♂	Clear/granular	↓↓	↑↑	↑↑	↑↑	↑	↓	↓
22	65	♂	Granular/clear	↓↓	↑	↑	↑	↑	↓	↓
23	42	♂	Chromophobic	↓↓	↑	↑	↑↑	↑↑	=	↓
24	65	♀	Clear/granular	↓↓	↑↑	↑↑	=	↑	↓	↓

↑ small increase; ↑↑ large increase; = no increase; ↓ small decrease; ↓↓ large decrease; *G6Pase*, glucose-6-phosphatase; *Syn*, glycogen synthase; *PHO*, glycogen phosphorylase; *G6PDH*, glucose-6-phosphate dehydrogenase; *GAPDH*, glyceraldehyde-3-phosphate dehydrogenase; *APase*, acid phosphatase; *GGT*, γ-glutamyltransferase

Oncocytic Tubules and Oncocytomas

A fourth type of epithelial kidney tumor which frequently appears in rats treated with NNM or a number of other chemicals is the oncocytoma (Bannasch et al. 1986b). This tumor type, which was described for the first time in man by Hamperl (1962), attracted great attention in the past two decades due to an apparently increasing incidence and a much more favorable prognosis than renal cell carcinomas (van der Walt 1983; Eble and Hull 1984; Zerban et al. 1987; Ortmann et al. 1988a, b). Like the human renal oncocytoma, the experimental oncocytoma grows very slowly and is considered benign (Bannasch et al. 1986b).

The ultrastructural equivalent of the characteristic light microscopical appearance of the renal oncocytes is an accumulation of atypical mitochondria (Fig. 6a) (Krech et al. 1981). It had been shown earlier that the rat renal oncocytoma derives from oncocytic tubules (Fig. 6b, c), involving distal parts of the tubular system (Bannasch et al. 1978a), but only in the last few years has Nogueira proved by careful light and electron microscopical studies that these tumors originate from the collecting duct system (Nogueira 1987; Nogueira and Bannasch 1988). In cooperation with the Department of Urology of the University of Heidelberg, Zerban and colleagues (1987) were able to show that human renal oncocytomas have exactly the same histogenesis, and this has since been confirmed by two other groups (Ortmann et al. 1988a, b; Störkel et al. 1988b).

Enzyme histochemical studies revealed that the oncocytic tubules and tumors induced with NNM in rats exhibit an increased activity of the mitochondrial enzyme succinate dehydrogenase, corresponding to the large number of mitochondria rich in cristae (Tsuda et al. 1986). Similarly, an increased content of the mitochondrial cytochrome-c-oxidase has been demonstrated in renal oncocytes of both man (Ortmann et al. 1988a, b) and rats (Mayer et al. 1989) by immunohistochemical procedures and has been recommended as a useful marker for the detection and differential diagnosis of oncocytomas. Of particular interest is that the activity of the glucose-6-phosphate dehydrogenase, the key enzyme of the pentose phosphate pathway, which is increased in most other types of renal cell tumors, is normal or decreased in the oncocytic lesions (Tsuda et al. 1986). This might explain the rarity of ribosomes and the slow growth of the oncocytic lesions.

A most intriguing observation in the animal model is the occasional appearance of tubules or microtumors which consist of both oncocytes

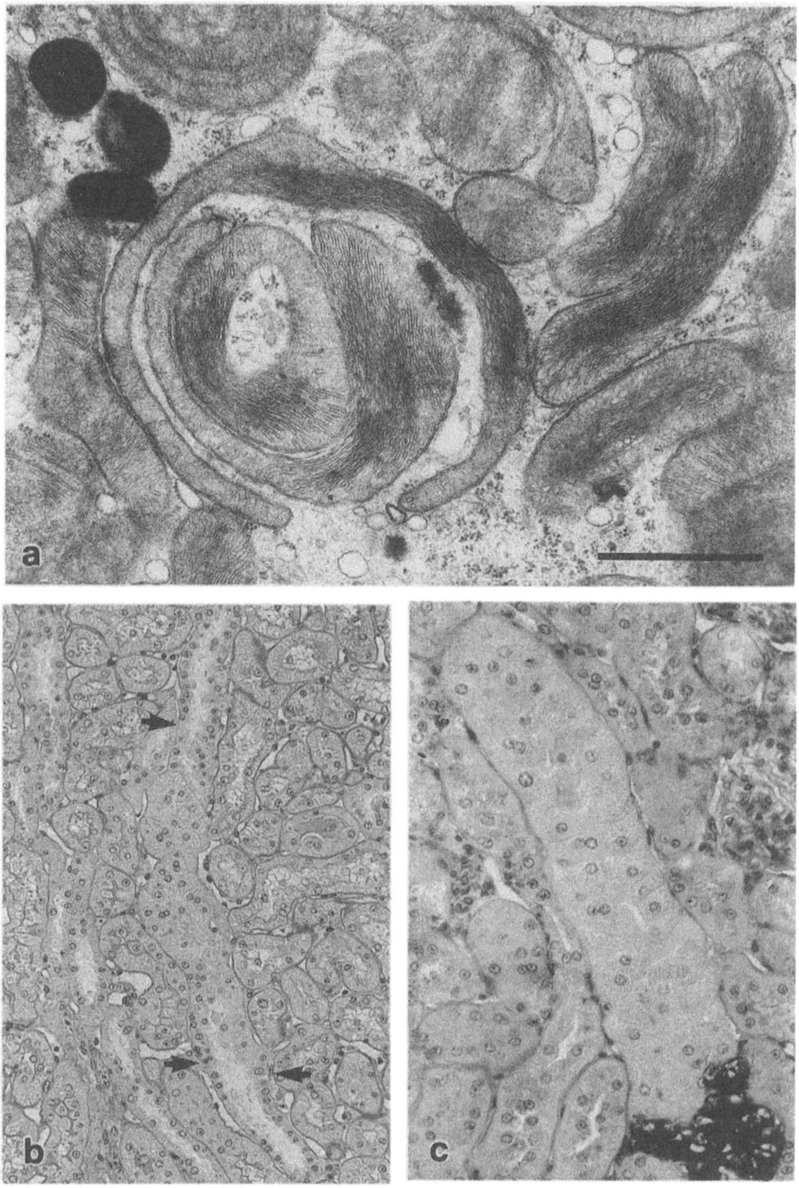

Fig. 6a–c. Oncocytic renal lesions induced in rat with *N*-nitrosomorpholine. **a** Portion of oncocyte crowded with atypical mitochondria containing abundant cristal membranes. Uranylacetate and lead citrate, TEM, ×25000. **b** Cortical collecting duct partly lined by oncocytes. Note transition (↓) of oncocytic portion to segments of normal appearance. Tri-PAS, ×160. **c** Altered renal tubule predominantly lined by oncocytes but also containing some (clear) cells storing glycogen (black) in excess as demonstrated by the PAS reaction. Tri-PAS, ×250

and clear cells storing glycogen in excess (Bannasch et al. 1978b; Nogueira and Bannasch 1989). Whereas this finding underlines the concept of a common histogenesis of both clear cell tumors and oncocytomas from the collecting duct system in the rat, it is difficult to understand the relationship between clear cells and oncocytes in view of the different prognosis of clear cell carcinomas and oncocytomas in man, which appears to correlate with characteristic cytogenetic and molecular genetic differences (Kovacs et al. 1989a). Even in more advanced rat renal oncocytomas small amounts of glycogen are often found (Bannasch et al. 1978b). As in many human oncocytomas of other sites, this glycogen is usually not located in the cytoplasmic matrix but is accumulated within atypical mitochondria. This finding suggests a peculiar disturbance of carbohydrate metabolism in the oncocytomas.

Conclusion

Recent studies on the pathobiology of renal carcinogenesis have revealed that this process is much more diverse than was anticipated some years ago (Bannasch and Zerban 1990). In addition to the proximal nephron, the collecting duct system has been established as a frequent site of origin of renal cell tumors. Instead of one type of renal cell carcinoma deriving from the cortex, as described by an international group in the WHO classification in 1981 (WHO 1981), several types of renal cell tumors have been separated in both laboratory animals and man. As to the mechanism of renal carcinogenesis, the experimental evidence strongly suggests that fundamental aberrations in the energy metabolism, which are most probably triggered by as yet unknown primary molecular alterations, play an essential role.

References

Bannasch P, Zerban H (1986) Renal cell adenoma and carcinoma, rat. In: Jones TC, Mohr U, Hunt RD (eds) Monographs on pathology of laboratory animals. Urinary system. Springer, Berlin Heidelberg New York Tokyo, pp 112–139

Bannasch P, Zerban H (1990) Animal models and renal carcinogenesis. In: Eble JN (ed) Tumors and tumor-like conditions of the kidney and ureters. Churchill Livingstone, New York, Edinburgh London Melbourne, pp 1–34

Bannasch P, Schacht U, Storch E (1974) Morphogenese und Mikromorphologie epithelialer Nierentumoren bei Nitrosomorpholin-vergifteten Ratten. I. Induktion und Histologie der Tumoren. Z Krebsforsch 81: 311–331
Bannasch P, Krech R, Zerban H (1978a) Morphogenese und Mikromorphologie epithelialer Nierentumoren bei Nitrosomorpholin-vergifteten Ratten. II. Tubuläre Glykogenose und die Genese von klar- oder acidophilzelligen Tumoren. Z Krebsforsch 92: 63–86
Bannasch P, Krech R, Zerban H (1978b) Morphogenese und Mikromorphologie epithelialer Nierentumoren bei Nitrosomorpholin-vergifteten Ratten. III. Onkocytentubuli und Onkocytome. Z Krebsforsch 92: 87–104
Bannasch P, Mayer D, Krech R (1979) Neoplastische und präneoplastische Veränderungen bei Ratten nach einmaliger oraler Applikation von N-Nitrosomorpholin. J Cancer Res Clin Oncol 94: 233–248
Bannasch P, Krech R, Zerban H (1980) Morphogenese und Mikromorphologie epithelialer Nierentumoren bei Nitrosomorpholin-vergifteten Ratten. IV. Tubuläre Läsionen und basophile Tumoren. J Cancer Res Clin Oncol 98: 243–265
Bannasch P, Hacker HJ, Tsuda H, Zerban H (1986a) Aberrant regulation of carbohydrate metabolism and metamorphosis during renal carcinogenesis. Adv Enzyme Regul 25: 279–296
Bannasch P, Zerban H, Hacker HJ (1986b) Oncocytoma, kidney, rat. In: Jones TC, Mohr U, Hunt RD (eds) Monographs on pathology of laboratory animals. Urinary system. Springer, Berlin Heidelberg New York Tokyo, pp 49–60
Bannasch P, Nogueira E, Zerban H, Beck K, Mayer D (1988) Sequential phenotypic conversion of renal epithelial cells during neoplastic development. In: Feo F, Pani P, Columbano A, Garcea R (eds) Chemical carcinogenesis. Plenum Publishing, pp 209–216
Bannasch P, Nogueira E, Zerban H (1989) Zytologie und Zytogenese experimenteller epithelialer Nierentumoren. Verh Dtsch Ges Pathol 73: 301–313
Beck K (1988) Induktion und Modulation der Entwicklung von Nierenzelltumoren der Ratte durch Streptozotocin und dessen diabetogenen Effekt. Thesis, Universität Heidelberg
Berger CS, Sandberg AA, Todd JAD, Pennington RD, Haddad FS, Hecht BK, Hecht F (1986) Chromosomes in kidney, ureter, and bladder cancer. Cancer Genet Cytogenet 23: 1–24
Carrol PR, Murty VVS, Reuter V, Ihanwar S, Fair WR, Whitmore WF, Chaganti RSK (1987) Abnormalities at chromosome region 3p 12–14 characterize clear cell renal carcinoma. Cancer Genet Cytogenet 26: 253–259
Dees JH, Reuber MD, Trump BF (1976) Adenocarcinoma of the kidney. I. Ultrastructure of renal adenocarcinomas induced in rats by N-(4′-fluoro-4-biphenylyl)-acetamide. J Natl Cancer Inst 57: 779–794
De Jong B, Oosterhuis JW, Idenburg VJS, Castedo SMMJ, Dam A, Mensink HJA: Cytogenetics of 12 cases of renal adenocarcinoma. Cancer Genet Cytogenet 30: 53–61
Eble JN (ed) (1990) Tumors and tumor-like conditions of the kidney and ureters. Churchill Livingstone, New York Edinburgh London Melbourne

Eble JN, Hull MT (1984) Morphologic features of renal oncocytoma: A light and electron microscopic study. Hum Pathol 15: 1054–1061
Grawitz P (1983) Die sogenannten Lipome der Niere. Virchows Arch 93: 39–63
Gusek W (1975) Die Ultrastruktur Cycasin-induzierter Nierenadenome. Virchows Arch [A] 365: 221–237
Hamperl H (1962) Onkocyten und Onkocytome. Virchows Arch [A] 335: 452–483
Hard GC (1986) Renal carcinogenesis, rat. In: Jones TC, Mohr U, Hunt RD (eds) Monographs on pathology of laboratory animals. Urinary system. Springer, Berlin Heidelberg New York Tokyo pp 45–49
Hard GC, Butler WH (1971a) Ultrastructural aspects of renal adenocarcinoma induced in the rat by dimethylnitrosamine. Cancer Res 31: 366–372
Hard GC, Butler WH (1971b) Morphogenesis of epithelial neoplasms induced in the rat kidney by dimethylnitrosamine. Cancer Res 31: 1496–1505
Heatfield BM, Hinton DE, Trump BF (1976) Adenocarcinoma of the kidney. II. Enzyme histochemistry of renal adenocarcinomas induced in rats by N-(4′-fluoro-4-biphenylyl)-acetamide. J Natl Cancer Inst 57: 795–808
Hiasa Y, Ito N (1987) Experimental induction of renal tumors. Crit Rev Toxicol 17: 279–343
Hruban Z, Mochizuki Y, Morris HP, Slesers A (1973) Ultrastructure of Morris renal tumors. J Natl Cancer Inst 50: 1487–1495
Hull MT, Eble JN (1987) Myelinoid lamellated cytoplamic inclusions in human renal adenocarcinomas: An ultrastructural study. Ultrastruct Pathol 12: 41–48
Ito N, Johno J, Marugami M, Konishi Y, Hiasa Y (1966) Histopathological and autoradiographic studies on kidney tumors induced by N-nitrosodimethylamine in rat. Gann 57: 595–604
Jasmin G, Riopelle JL (1969) Transplantation de trois tumeurs rénales induites chez le rat par la diméthylnitrosamine. Int J Cancer 4: 299–311
Kovacs G (1990) Application of molecular cytogenetic techniques to the evaluation of renal parenchymal tumors. J Cancer Res Clin Oncol 116: 318–323
Kovacs G, Frisch S (1989) Clonal chromosome abnormalities in tumor cells from patients with sporadic renal cell carcinomas. Cancer Res 49: 651–659
Kovacs G, Welter C, Wilkins L, Blin N, DeRiese W (1989a) Renal oncocytoma. A phenotypic and genotypic entity of renal parenchymal tumors. Am J Pathol 134: 967–971
Kovacs G, Wilkens L, Papp T, DeRiese W (1989b) Differentiation between papillary and nonpapillary renal cell carcinomas by DNA analysis. J Natl Cancer Inst 81: 527–530
Krech R, Zerban H, Bannasch P (1981) Mitochondrial anomalies in renal oncocytes induced in rat by N-nitrosomorpholine. Eur J Cell Biol 25: 331–339
Krech R, Fonatsch C, Peters B, Löhrs U (1989) Morphologie und Wachstumsfraktion von Nierenzellkarzinomen des Menschen in Korrelation zu zytogenetischen Daten. Verh Dtsch Ges Pathol 73: 409–414
Lipsky MM Jr, Trump BF (1988) Chemically induced renal epithelial neoplasia in experimental animals. Int Rev Exp Pathol 30: 357–383

Mao P, Molnar JJ (1967) The fine structure and histochemistry of lead-induced renal tumors in rats. Am J Pathol 50: 571–603
Mayer D, Bannasch P (1988) Activity of glycogen synthase and phosphorylase and glucose-6-phosphate content in renal clear cell carcinomas. J Cancer Res Clin Oncol 114: 369–372
Mayer D, Weber E, Kadenbach B, Bannasch P (1989) Immunocytochemical demonstration of cytochrome c oxidase as a marker for renal oncocytes and oncocytomas. Toxicol Pathol 17: 46–49
McGiven AR, Ireton HJ (1972) Renal epithelial dysplasia and neoplasia in rats given dimethylnitrosamine. J Pathol 108: 187–190
Merkow LP, Epstein SM, Slifkin M, Pardo M (1973) The ultrastructure of renal neoplasms induced by aflatoxin B_1. Cancer Res 33: 1608–1614
Nogueira E (1987) Rat renal carcinogenesis after chronic simultaneous exposure to lead acetate and N-nitrosodiethylamine. Virchows Arch [B] 53: 365–374
Nogueira E, Bannasch P (1988) Cellular origin of rat renal oncocytoma. Lab Invest 59: 337–343
Nogueira E, Klimek F, Weber E, Bannasch P (1989) Origin of renal clear cell tumors from the collecting duct. Virchows Arch [B] 57: 275–283
Oberling C, Rivière M, Haguenau F (1960) Ultrastructure of clear cells in renal carcinoma and its importance for the demonstration of their renal origin. Nature 186: 402–403
Ortmann M, Vierbuchen M, Fischer R (1988a) Renal oncocytoma. II. Lectin- and immunohistochemical features indicating an origin from the collecting duct. Virchows Arch [B] 56: 175–184
Ortmann M, Vierbuchen M, Koller G, Fischer R (1988b) Renal oncocytoma. I. Cytochrome c oxidase in normal and neoplastic renal tissue as detected by immunohistochemistry – a valuable aid to distinguish oncocytomas from renal cell carcinomas. Virchows Arch [B] 56: 165–173
Störkel SB, Pannen B, Thoenes W, Steart PV, Wagner S, Drenckhahn D (1988a) Intercalated cells as a probable source for the development of renal oncocytoma. Virchows Arch [B] 56: 185–189
Störkel S, Steart PV, Drenckhahn D, Thoenes W (1988b) The human chromophobe cell renal carcinoma – its probable relation to intercalated cells of the collecting duct. Virchows Arch [B] 56: 237–245
Teyssier JR, Henry I, Dozier C, Ferre D, Adnet JJ, Pluot M (1986) Recurrent deletion of the short arm of chromosome 3 in human renal cell carcinoma: shift of the c-raf 1 locus. J Natl Cancer Inst 77: 1187–1195
Thoenes W, Störkel S, Rumpelt H-J (1985) Human chromophobe cell renal carcinoma. Virchows Arch [B] 48: 207–217
Thoenes W, Störkel S, Rumpelt H-J (1986) Histopathology and classification of renal cell tumors (adenomas, oncocytomas, and carcinomas). The basic cytological and histopathological elements and their use for diagnostics. Pathol Res Pract 181: 125–143
Thoenes W, Störkel S, Rumpelt H-J, Moll R, Baum HP, Werner S (1988) Chromophobe cell renal carcinoma and its variants – a report on 32 cases. J Pathol 155: 277–287
Tsuda H, Hacker HJ, Katayama H, Masui T, Ito N, Bannasch P (1985) Correlative histochemical studies on preneoplastic and neoplastic lesions in the kidney of rats treated with nitrosamines. Virchows Arch [B] 51: 385–404

Van der Walt JD, Reid HAS, Risdon RA, Shaw HF (1983) Renal oncocytoma. A review of the literature and report of an unusual multicentric case. Virchows Arch [A] 398: 291–304

Weber G (1980) Enzymic programs of human renal adenocarcinoma. In: Sufrin G, Beckley SA (eds) Renal adenocarcinoma. UICC Publications, Geneva, pp 44–50

WHO (1981) International histological classification of tumours. In: Mostofi FK, Sesterhenn JA, Sobin LH (eds) Histological typing of kidney tumours, Vol 25

Yoshida MA, Ohyashiki K, Ochi H, Gibas Z, Pontes JE, Prout GR, Sandberg AA (1986) Cytogenetic studies of tumor tissue from patients with nonfamilial renal cell carcinomas. Cancer Res 46: 2139–2147

Zerban H, Nogueira E, Riedasch G, Bannasch P (1987) Renal oncocytoma: origin from the collecting duct. Virchows Arch [B] 52: 375–387

Molecular Analysis of DNA Sequences on Chromosome 3 in Patients with Renal Cell Carcinoma

H. Brauch[1], K. Tory[2], S. Hosoe[2], P. Anglard[3], M. Lerman[2], M. Linehan[3], and B. Zbar[2]

Introduction

Analyses of human tumor karyotypes have revealed that tumors display chromosomal aberrations [12]. A modern view of carcinogenesis suggests that cancer is a genetic disease. In this article we describe the theory on which this view is based and the technique to identify genetic changes on a molecular level. We applied both theory and technique to human renal cell carcinoma in order to understand genetic mechanisms involved in the origin of this neoplasm.

The Two Mutation Theory of Cancer

The two mutation theory by A. Knudson [6] explains the origin of cancer by as few as two mutations in a cell and is based on epidemiological, molecular and clinical studies. Mathematical analysis of age of occurrence in hereditary and nonhereditary forms of both retinoblastoma and Wilms' tumor suggested that two mutations were required to produce these cancers. D.E. Comings [4] refined this theory by pointing out that both mutations must affect homologous loci. As a consequence of such homologous mutations, function of both copies of a gene is lost. This gene should be important for normal differentiation of cells and therefore should have a tumor-suppressing acti-

[1] Present address: Deutsches Krebsforschungszentrum, Institut für Experimentelle Pathologie, Im Neuenheimer Feld 280, W-6900 Heidelberg 1, FRG
[2] National Cancer Institute – Frederick Cancer Research Facility, Laboratory of Immunobiology, Frederick, MD 21702, USA
[3] National Cancer Institute, Urologic Oncology Section, Surgery Branch, Bethesda, MD 20892, USA

G. Staehler S. Pomer (Eds.)
Basic and Clinical Research on Renal Cell Carcinoma

vity. Genes which are involved in tumorigenesis and can be inactivated by a recessive mechanism are called tumor suppressor genes.

The two mutation theory allows us to explain hereditary and nonhereditary tumors by the same mechanism of inactivation (Fig. 1). In hereditary tumors the first mutation runs in the germline and is already present in sperm or ovum before fertilization. This single mutation is not sufficient to produce cancer but must be followed by a somatic mutation later in life. Both mutations together produce cancer. In nonhereditary tumors both mutations are somatic mutations acquired after fertilization. According to this theory both hereditary and nonhereditary forms of cancer follow the same mechanism of inactivation of alleles but differ in their time course. Hereditary tumors have an early age of onset because only a single somatic mutation needs to be acquired. Nonhereditary tumors usually occur in the second half of life, since it takes longer to acquire two somatic mutations consecutively.

Detection of Genetic Changes by Restriction Fragment Length Polymorphism Analysis of Normal and Tumor DNA

Traditionally, genetic changes have been detected by cytogenetic analyses of human tumor karyotypes. On a molecular level, subtle genetic changes can be detected by DNA polymorphism analysis [2]. DNA polymorphisms are normal, heritable variations in DNA sequence. Each individual inherits one set of chromosomes from the mother and the other set of chromosomes from the father. These homologous chromosomes from father and mother can differ. Such differences are based on a variable number of restriction sites for bacterial restriction enzymes. These are constant restriction sites which are always present at a locus, on each chromosome and consequently in each individual. There are also variable restriction sites, which may or may not be present. Due to these variable restriction sites individuals differ in the constitution of such loci.

Normal and tumor DNA was subjected to restriction fragment length polymorphism (RFLP) analysis [3]. DNA was extracted from blood and tumor tissue and subjected to restriction with bacterial restriction enzyme; fragments were separated according to size during agarose gel electrophoresis and blotted to a nylon membrane. After hybridization with a radiolabeled homologous DNA sequence specifically recognizing that locus, polymorphic bands were visualized after

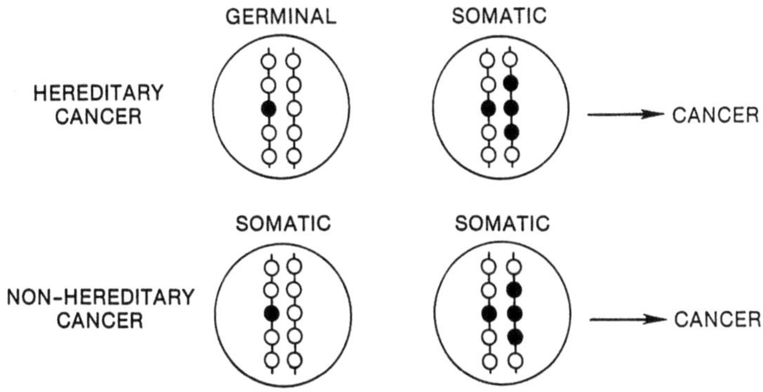

Fig. 1. The two mutation theory of cancer. Every cell in the body of an individual contains a pair of genes at homologous loci, which may predispose this individual to cancer. Tumors develop after mutation at both homologous loci as a result of loss of normal gene function. Mutations are indicated as black circles. There are hereditary and nonhereditary forms of cancer. They share the same mechanism of inactivation but differ in their time course. Individuals with an inherited predisposition for cancer carry one mutation in the germline which will be followed by a somatic mutation after fertilization. In patients with nonhereditary cancer the wild-type alleles are lost both by somatic mutations after fertilization (From Zbar et al. [13], with permission)

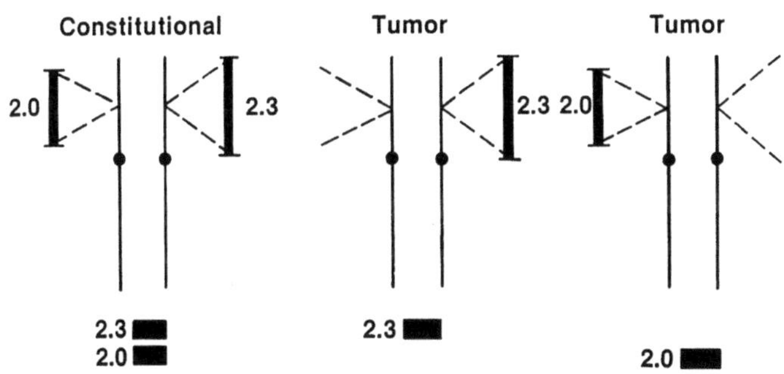

Fig. 2. Scheme of DNA polymorphism and detection of genetic changes in tumors by restriction fragment length polymorphism analysis. A locus on a pair of homologous loci is enlarged. The constitutional DNA depicted is heterozygous as a result of a difference in DNA sequence in one chromosome. Hypothetical Southern blot analysis and hybridization with a DNA specific probe visualizes this polymorphism as two bands of different size. The larger 2.3 kb band will be originated from the right chromosome cut out in between two constant restriction sites. The smaller fragment of 2.0 kb will be originated from the left chromosome and is due to an additional variable restriction site. The residual 0.3 kb piece is cut off and cannot be detected. In tumors from patients with heterozygous constitutional genotype, loss of alleles can be determined. By comparison of constitutional and tumor genotype there is only one allele present in the tumor DNA. Either one of the alleles may be lost in sporadic tumors (From Zbar et al. [13], with permission)

autoradiography. There are homozygous individuals, both of whose chromosomes contain the same number of restriction sites, either constant or constant plus variable. These individuals fail to be informative in loss of heterozygosity studies, because each signal is the sum of two chromosomal fragments. Heterozygous individuals are those who carry two different chromosomes with respect to restriction sites (Fig. 2). A heterozygous individual has one chromosome with only constant restriction sites and another chromosome with constant restriction sites plus an additional variable site. In Southern blot analysis these alleles can be separated because they differ in size. Each allele now represents the chromosome of its origin. This heterozygous constitution represents an informative situation which allows determination of loss of heterozygosity in DNA of tumors. Furthermore, this powerful technique allows us to assess parental origin of a particular chromosome upon haplotype analysis. This is the prerequisite for determining whether a specific DNA sequence deleted in a tumor qualifies for harboring a tumor suppressor gene.

Deletion of Sequences on the Short Arm of Chromosome 3 in Sporadic Renal Cell Carcinoma

Karyotype analysis of renal cell carcinomas showed that chromosome 3 is the prime target for a genetic change in these tumors. This change was cytogenetically defined as a deletion on the short arm of chromosome 3 [7]. We subjected 60 sporadic renal cell carcinomas to RFLP analysis, comparing normal DNA with tumor DNA at 3p loci. Figure 3 gives an example of such an analysis. The locus analyzed is DNF15S2 detected by the probe pH3H2 which detects a *Hin*dIII polymorphism. This polymorphism consists of two alleles with the size 2.3 kb and 2.0 kb. Comparison of tumor versus normal DNA showed that one allele is lost in these tumors. In these sporadic renal cell carcinomas either one of the two alleles can be lost. Loss of heterozygosity is shown as a reduction in signal intensity. Remaining signal is due to a contamination of normal cells in the primary tumor tissue. In patient 15, allele 1 completely disappeared after the tumor was passaged through a nude mouse, selecting for tumor cells. Tumors could also be cleaned up by extraction with magnetic-bead-bound monoclonal antibodies directed to lymphocyte surface antigens [8]. Altogether we tested for loss of heterozygosity at ten 3p loci, which are distributed over the entire length of the short arm of chromosome 3. Of the 60 patients, 58 were informative and 51 (88%) showed loss

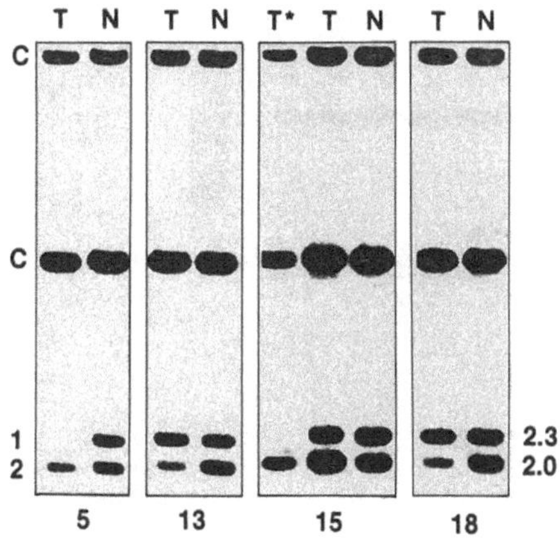

Fig. 3. Loss of heterozygosity at the DNF15S2 locus on the short arm of chromosome 3 in patients with sporadic renal cell carcinoma. The *panel* shows autoradiographs of Southern blot filters. DNA was isolated from individual renal cell carcinomas and normal lymphocytes, digested with *Hin*dIII, fractionated on agarose gel electrophoresis, and transferred to nylon filters. After hybridization with radiolabeled pH3H2, the probe detects two constant bands (*C*) and two polymorphic bands, allele 1 (2.3 kb) and allele 2 (2.0 kb). For each patient normal and tumor DNA was compared. The constitutional DNA (*N*) of patients 5, 13, 15 and 18 was heterozygous. In their tumor DNA (*T*) one of the two polymorphic alleles was lost. This loss shows as a reduction in signal intensity. Residual signal was due to contamination with normal tumor infiltrated lymphocytes. For patient 15 the renal tumor was grown in a nude mouse (*T**) resulting in purification of the tumor cells and total loss of allele 1 after one passage (From Zbar et al. [14], with permission)

of heterozygosity at one or more loci. In most cases loss of 3p alleles was consistent with a terminal deletion. There were six exceptions in which some of the 3p loci were retained in the tumor (Fig. 4). By comparison, a common region deleted in these tumors is bounded by the loci D3S2 and D3S22 [1]. This region extends from 3p21 to 3p26 and contains two loci which genetically link to von Hippel-Lindau disease [5, 10].

Implication of Loss of 3p Alleles in Tumors of Patients with von Hippel-Lindau Disease

Von Hippel-Lindau disease is an autosomal dominant trait which predisposes patients to developing retinal angiomas, cerebellar- and

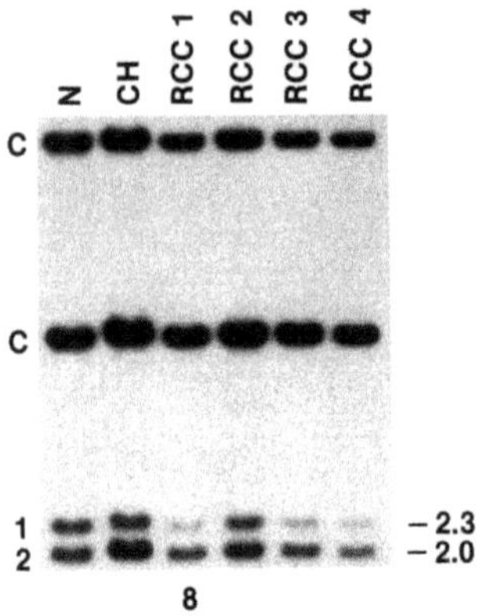

Fig. 4. Restriction fragment length polymorphism analysis at the DNF15S2 locus in tumors of a patient with von Hippel-Lindau disease. The *panel* shows autoradiographs of Southern blot filters. DNA was isolated from four discrete renal cell carcinomas of left and right kidney, one cerebellar hemangioblastoma and corresponding normal kidney, digested with *Hin*dIII, fractionated on agarose gel electrophoresis and transferred to nylon filters. After hybridization with radiolabelled pH3H2 the patient's constitutional DNA (*N*) was heterozygous for allele 1 (2.3 kb) and allele 2 (2.0 kb). In four renal cell carcinomas (*RCC1–RCC4*), as well as in one cerebellar hemangioblastoma (*CH*), the same allele, allele 1, was lost (From Tory et al. [11], with permission)

spinal hemangioblastomas, pheochromocytomas, renal cell carcinoma and benign tumors of the epididymis and pancreas [9]. Genetic linkage of the disease allele was described for the 3p loci *RAF1* [10] and D3S18 [5]. If von Hippel-Lindau disease represents a hereditary form of renal cell carcinoma, 3p RFLP analyses of renal cell carcinomas of patients with von Hippel-Lindau disease should give an indication of whether or not these tumors arise as a consequence of inactivation of a tumor suppressor gene. As outlined earlier in the two mutation theory of tumorigenesis, RFLP analyses in patients with a hereditary disease allow us to discriminate between two homologous alleles in their tumors, and test for a recessive mechanism of inactivation.

The following predictions were made for tumors of patients with von Hippel-Lindau disease:

1. Renal cell carcinoma of patients with von Hippel-Lindau disease should have a 3p deletion.
2. Since patients with von Hippel-Lindau disease often have multiple tumors, this deletion should be the same in all tumors.
3. The allele lost in the tumors should be the wild type allele.

4. The allele retained in the tumor should be the allele coinherited with the chromosome carrying the germline defect responsible for von Hippel-Lindau disease.

Figure 4 illustrates the results obtained by RFLP analysis of four renal cell carcinomas and a cerebellar hemangioblastoma of a patient with von Hippel-Lindau disease. The patient's normal DNA was informative at the 3p locus DNF15S2. In all tumors there was loss of heterozygosity, and the same allele, allele 1, was deleted. Parental origin of the alleles, and the father's blood DNA, was determined in the analysis (not shown); the affected mother was deceased. Allele 1 was inherited from the unaffected father. This allele, therefore, represented the wild type allele which was lost in all von Hippel-Lindau tumors of the son. Allele 2 must have been inherited from the affected mother, together with the disease allele. This allele was retained in all tumors. Similar results were obtained in multiple renal cell carcinomas and other tumors of seven von Hippel-Lindau patients (not shown). The presence of the disease allele in the tumors gives indirect evidence for a preceeding germline mutation which was followed by the loss of the wild type allele.

Conclusions

Renal cell carcinoma, sporadic and hereditary, is characterized by loss of alleles on the short arm of chromosome 3. The deleted area harbors loci which genetically link to the von Hippel-Lindau disease gene. This gene follows a recessive mechanism of inactivation in renal cell carcinoma and other tumors of patients with von Hippel-Lindau disease. It therefore fulfills criteria for a tumor suppressor gene, and is involved in the development of tumors of von Hippel-Lindau disease, but we cannot yet be certain whether it is the same as the gene involved in the development of sporadic renal cell carcinomas.

References

1. Anglard P, Tory K, Brauch H, et al. (1991) Molecular analysis of genetic changes in the origin and development of renal cell carcinoma. Cancer Research 51: 1071–1077.
2. Barker D, Schafer M, White R (1984) Restriction sites containing CpG show a higher frequency of polymorphisms in human DNA. Cell 36: 131–138

3. Brauch H, Johnson B, Hovis J, et al. (1987) Molecular analysis of the short arm of chromosome 3 in small-cell and non-small-cell carcinoma of the lung. N Engl J M 317: 1109–1113
4. Comings DE (1973) A general theory of carcinogenesis. Proc Natl Acad Sci USA 70: 3324–3328
5. Hosoe S, Brauch H, Latif F, et al. (1990) Localization of the von Hippel-Lindau disease gene to a small region of chromosome 3. Genomics 8: 634–640
6. Knudson AG Jr (1972) Mutation and Cancer: a model for Wilms' tumor of the kidney. J Nat Cancer Inst 48: 313–324
7. Kovacs G, Szücs S, De Riese W, Baumgärtl H (1987) Specific chromosome aberration in human renal cell carcinoma. Int J Cancer 40: 171–178
8. Linehan M, Miller E, Anglard P, Merino M, Zbar B (1989) Improved detection of allele loss in renal cell carcinomas after removal of leucocytes by immunologic selection. J Natl Cancer Inst 81: 287–290
9. Melmon KL, Rosen S (1964) Lindau's Disease. Review of the literature and study of a large kindred. Am J Med 36: 595–617
10. Seizinger BR, Rouleau GS, Ozelius LJ, et al. (1988) Von Hippel-Lindau disease maps to the region of chromosome 3 associated with renal cell carcinoma. Nature 332: 268–269
11. Tory K, Brauch H, Linehan M, et al. (1989) Specific genetic change in tumors associated with von Hippel-Lindau disease. J Natl Cancer Inst 81: 1097–1101
12. Yunis JJ (1983) The chromosomal basis of human neoplasia. Science 221: 227–236
13. Zbar B (1989) Chromosomal deletions in lung cancer and renal cancer. In: DeVita VT, Jr., Hellmann S, Rosenberg SA (eds) Important Advances in Oncology. JB Lippincott Co, Philadelphia (PA)
14. Zbar B, Brauch H, Talmadge C, Linehan M (1988) Loss of alleles of loci on the short arm of chromosome 3 in renal cell carcinoma. Nature 327: 721–724

Cell Proliferation and Cellular Heterogeneity in Renal Cell Carcinoma

^{31}P NMR Spectroscopy of Human Tumor Cells In Vitro and In Vivo: Prospects for Applications to Renal Cell Carcinoma

W.E. Hull[1], A.C. Kuesel[1], and S. Pomer[2]

The Nuclear Magnetic Resonance Phenomenon

Many natural isotopes have a nuclear spin and can be induced to give radio frequency (RF), nuclear magnetic resonance (NMR) signals in a strong, applied magnetic field B_0. Important isotopes for biological NMR applications are listed in Table 1 along with their abundance, resonance frequency and relative detection sensitivity. The abundant isotope of carbon, ^{12}C, has no nuclear spin; the low sensitivity for ^{13}C means that labeling of substances will be necessary for biological applications.

The exact resonance frequencies for a given isotope are sensitive to the local molecular structure. These effects, called "chemical shifts", are in the Hz to KHz range and are expressed in ppm relative to a chosen reference signal. It is important to note that:

- An NMR spectrum is a fingerprint for chemical structure, i.e., the position and form of the signals can be used to identify molecular species.
- Mixtures can be analyzed without chromatographic separation; the area under a signal (integral) is proportional to the concentration of the substance.
- Signal linewidths contain information about molecular mobility and chemical exchange rates.
- Here it is very important to realize that linewidths are proportional to molecular weight; *macromolecules and tightly bound*

[1] Deutsches Krebsforschungszentrum, Abteilung Zentrale Spektroskopie, Im Neuenheimer Feld 280, W-6900 Heidelberg 1, FRG
[2] Chirurgische Universtätsklinik, Abteilung Urologie, Im Neuenheimer Feld 110, W-6900 Heidelberg 1, FRG

G. Staehler S. Pomer (Eds.)
Basic and Clinical Research on Renal Cell Carcinoma

Table 1. Important isotopes for biological NMR applications

Isotope	Abundance	Resonance frequency at 11.7 T	Relative sensitivity
^{1}H	100(%)	500 MHz	100
^{19}F	100	470	83
^{31}P	100	202	7
^{13}C	1.1	125	0.02

metabolites will normally not be detected or at best seen as a very broad background signal.
- Higher magnetic fields improve signal resolution and detection sensitivity.

It is of particular interest that the NMR technique is *nondestructive* and can be applied in a *noninvasive* manner in vivo.

Technically, NMR signals can be generated and manipulated in various ways to provide:

- Purely chemical/structural information (spectroscopy)
- Purely spatial information (imaging)
- Both chemical and spatial information (localized spectroscopy)

NMR in Cancer Research

There are many possibilities for the application of NMR spectroscopy, either purely as an analytical technique or for more biologically oriented problems:

- Detailed characterization and quantitation of individual metabolites
- Elucidation of enzyme mechanisms and metabolic pathways
- Investigation of processes involved in stimulation, malignant transformation and growth
- Monitoring the effects of hormones, cytokines, drugs and other therapies

The NMR techniques used and their applications can be classified as in vitro or in vivo. *In-vitro* or high-resolution, $B_0 = 2\text{–}14\,T$:

- Homogeneous solutions, cellular extracts
- Biologic fluids: urine, plasma, bile, CSF (0.3–1.5 ml)
- Solid tissue, biopsies (4°C, 0.1–1 g)

- Cell suspensions (10^6–10^8 cells)
- Perfused cells in a bioreactor or gel matrix

In-vivo, B_0 = 2–9 T (animal), 1–4 T (human)

- Use of surface coil techniques (best detection sensitivity) to study localized superficial tumors, e.g., human xenografts on nude mice
- More general imaging and image-guided spectroscopic techniques for internal organs (poor sensitivity)

Some typical applications for the different isotopes are:

^{1}H: all molecules, metabolic fingerprinting
^{13}C: metabolic pathways using labeled precursors
^{19}F: fluorine-containing antimetabolites, e.g., fluoropyrimidines, fluoro-sugars
^{31}P: monitor phosphate, nucleotides, phosphoesters for intracellular pH, energy status, phospholipid metabolism, respectively

The strategy we employ at the German Cancer Research Center is to combine in vitro and in vivo techniques at the highest possible field strengths to obtain high quality, detailed biochemical data which can provide a solid foundation for developing *useful* applications of in vivo NMR under the limitations of the clinical environment.

High-field ^{31}P NMR of Tumor Cells and Solid Tumors

^{31}P NMR is of particular interest for tumor cells since they can differ from normal cells in pH, energy metabolism and phospholipid turnover (proliferation rate). Human tumor cells can be studied as cultures in an appropriate matrix or as solid tumors (xenografts) in the nude mouse.

Methods

1. *In-vitro NMR at 11.7 T (202 MHz)*. Typically 2–8 × 10^7 cultured cells are harvested and mixed 1:1 with basement membrane gel (BMG; Matrigel EHS, Serva) and extruded as threads 250 μm in diameter which can be coiled into a compact form and perfused (1 ml/min) in a 10-mm NMR sample tube. This allows:

- Complete control of medium, additives, pH, temperature and, oxygen
- Continuous monitoring over several days with a time resolution of 30–60 min for individual spectra
  NMR data acquisition parameters used were: 12 μS RF pulse for a 45° nutation angle, and a 2 s repetition time; 1800 or 3600 transients were accumulated over 1 or 2 h.

2. *In vivo NMR at 7 T (121 MHz)*. Human tumor cell lines as xenografts (s.c. or i.m.) in nude mice can be examined at diameters of 1–3 cm using a 14-mm surface coil for localized spectroscopy. We can perform long-term, repetitive and noninvasive measurements without anesthetics to follow growth and therapy. Parameters used were: RF pulse of 8–32 μs, depending on the desired penetration depth for the detected volume; 2 s repetition time, 600 or 1200 transients in 20 or 40 min.

Results

Figures 1 and 2 compare the ^{1}H-decoupled ^{31}P NMR spectra of various human tumor cell lines as cell cultures under constant conditions and as xenografts. EJ-28 is a bladder carcinoma which forms cysts in vivo, MRI-H-186 and HeLa are cervix carcinomas, LX-1 is an axillary metastasis from a lung carcinoma, and CX-1 is a colon carcinoma. Each peak in a spectrum represents a particular type or class of phosphorus atom with a specific molecular environment. The assignments are as follows: NTP α, β, γ are the three phosphates of all nucleoside-5′-triphosphates (ATP, UTP, etc., cannot be separately resolved); NDPN are all dinucleotides of the NAD type; NDP-Hex are all nucleotide hexoses such as UDPG; PCr is phosphocreatine (used as chemical shift reference = 0 ppm), P_i is inorganic phosphate, either extracellular *e* (1 m*M* in medium) or intracellular *i*. Phosphomonoesters fall in the chemical shift range of 6–8, and the predominant species are phosphocholine (PC) and phosphoethanolamine (PE). The phosphodiesters appear at 2–4 ppm, and typically only glycero-3-phosphocholine (GPC) and glycero-3-phosphoethanolamine (GPE) are at detectable levels (>0.2 m*M*). CDP-choline (CDP-Cho) is normally detected only in EJ-28, which is also atypical in the absence of PCr. CDP-Cho can be detected in other cell lines when the pH of the medium is lowered to below 6.6.

P_i and the phosphomonoesters have pH-dependent chemical shifts that, with appropriate calibration, can be used to determine the intracellular pH_{int} to an accuracy of ca. 0.05 unit. In Fig. 1 all cultures show pH_{int} of 7.1 ± 0.1. The cell types have been ordered from bottom to top according to increasing PE. Although NTP phosphate signals represent 35% ± 5% of total phosphate in all cell types, the levels of PCr and the phospholipid metabolites vary in quite dramatic and characteristic ways.

Figure 2 shows that the corresponding xenografts also show significant differences in their phospholipid metabolites. Compared with

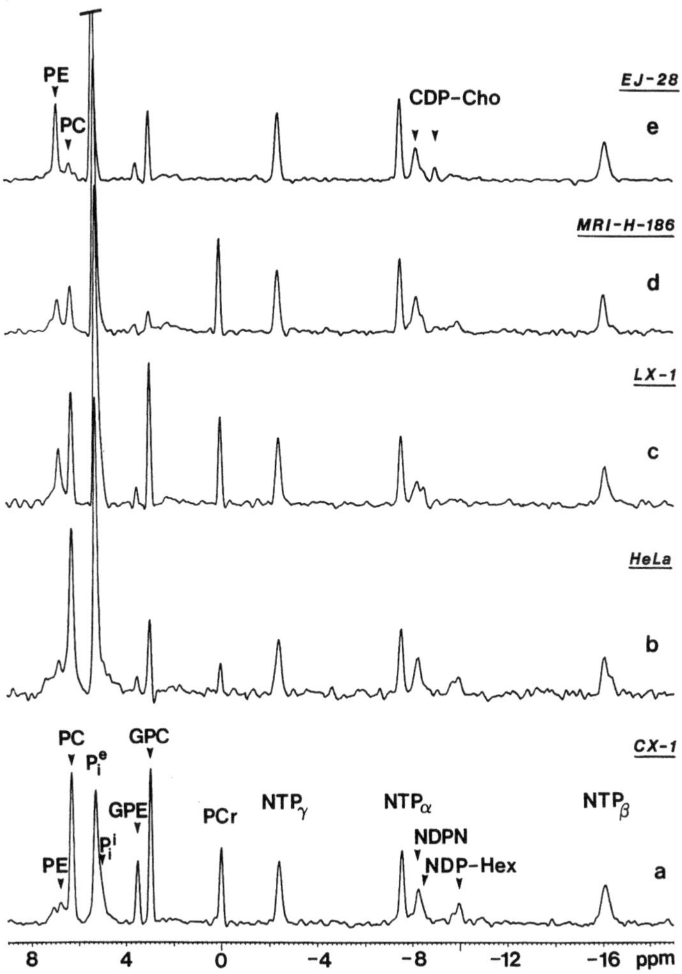

Fig. 1. ^{31}P NMR at 11.7 T (2 h acquisition). Human tumor cell lines cultured in basement membrane gel and perfused with Ham's F12, pH 7.3, 37 °C

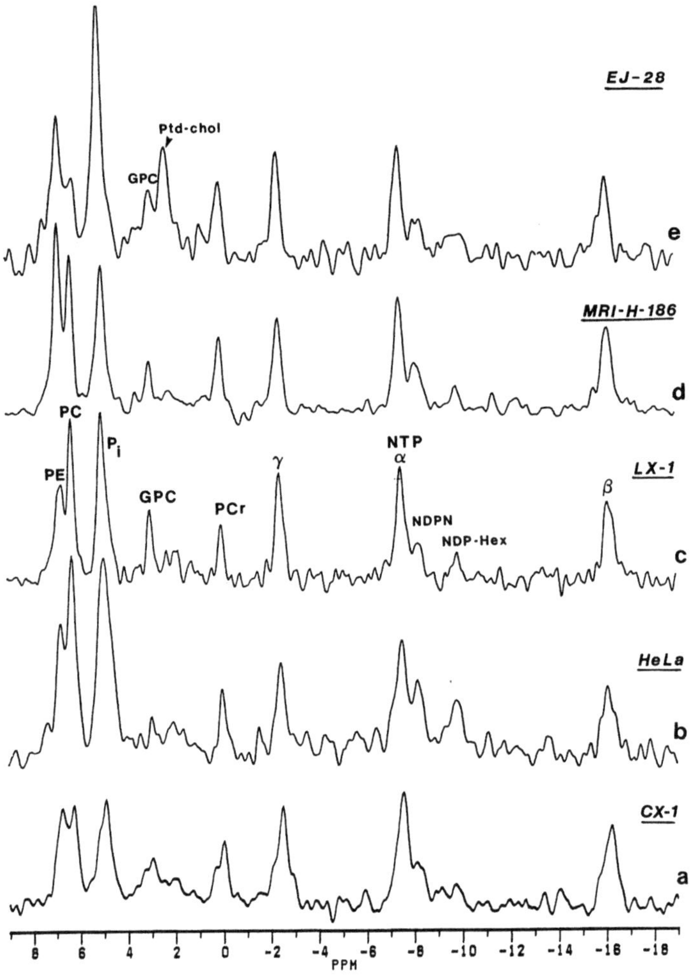

Fig. 2. In vivo ^{31}P NMR (7 T, 20 min). Human tumor cell lines as xenografts on nude mice

the cultured cells in perfusion we generally find higher levels of PE in vivo when it is low in culture. This is probably due to the absence of ethanolamine and the presence of choline in the medium used.

The in vitro culture spectra show better resolution and signal-to-noise as a result of the higher field strength used and the more homogeneous nature of the sample.

Figures 3 and 4 present our first results with a renal cell carcinoma (RCC) line established in the tumor bank of the German Cancer

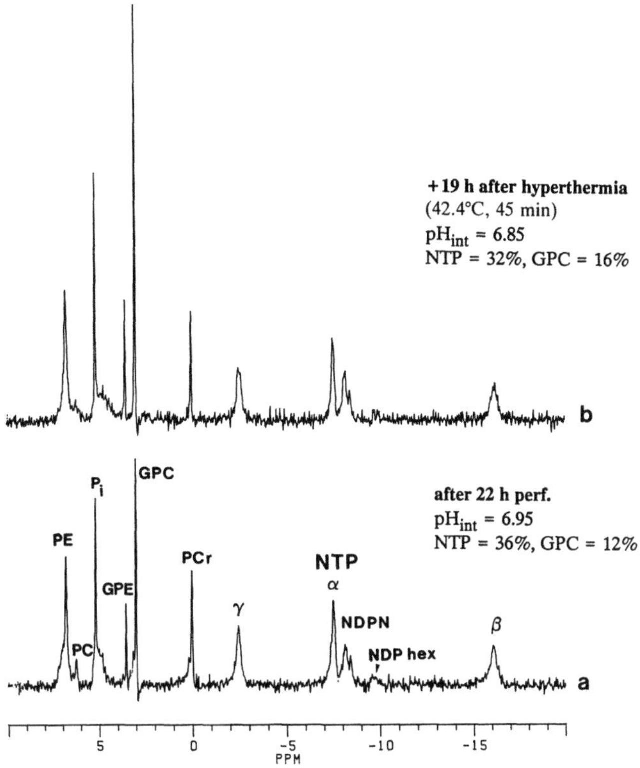

Fig. 3. ^{31}P NMR at 11.7 T (2 h acquisition). KTCTL-26A cell line, renal cell carcinoma (clear cell), in basement membrane gel perfused with Ham's F12, pH 7.3, 37 °C

Center. The perfusion was carried out under the same conditions as for Fig. 1. The sharp P_i resonance in Fig. 3a is from the medium (1 m*M*); the broader intracellular P_i signal shifted slightly to the right in the spectrum indicates a pH_{int} of 6.9–7.0 after 22 h in the spectrometer. The cells were subjected to a hyperthermia treatment, but there was little change in metabolism immediately or after 19 h (Fig. 3b). In Fig. 4, dramatic effects could be seen for treatment with recombinant interferon α-2b (Intron A, Essex Pharma) that was added to the perfusion medium. PCr and NTP levels drop; NDP and NMP can be detected. PE decreases and broadens and intracellular P_i broadens, indicating lower and heterogeneous pH_{int} (mean values are shown). The broad resonance under the GPC, GPE peaks (Fig. 4c) is suggestive of phospholipid debris (signals from intact phospholipid bilayers cannot be detected, Fig. 4a).

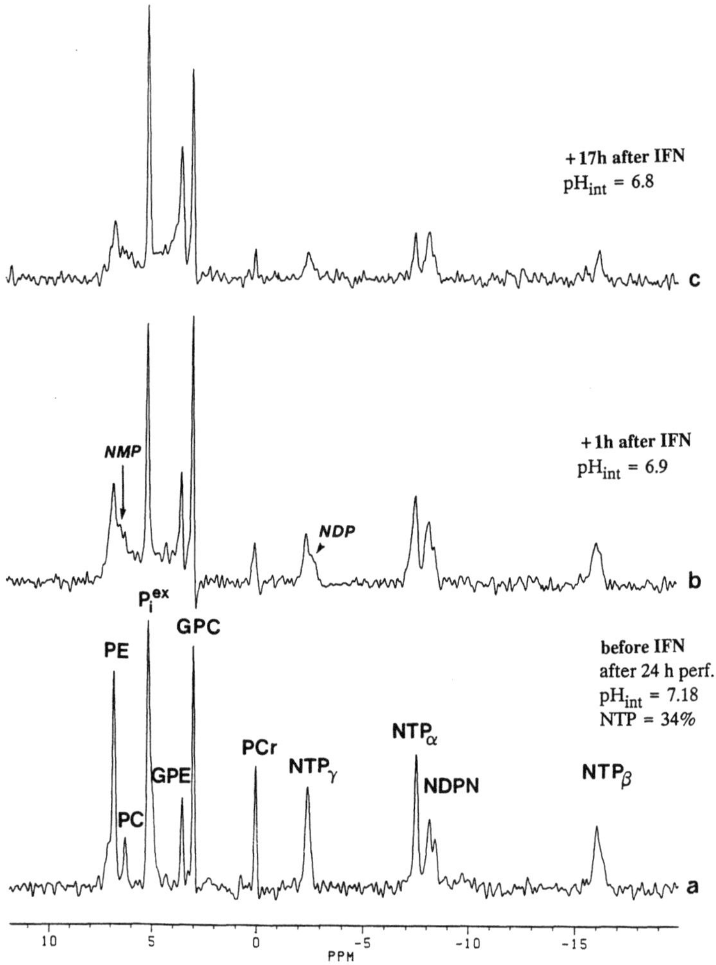

Fig. 4. ^{31}P NMR at 11.7 T (1 h acquisition). KTCL-26A cell line, renal cell carcinoma (clear cell), in basement membrane gel perfused with Ham's F12, pH 7.3, 37°C + interferon α-2b 5 × 10^6 units/300 mL

For in vivo studies a brain metastasis from a RCC patient was established as a xenograft in several nude mice. Figure 5 shows spectra from one such tumor (ca. 10 weeks after implantation) that had a reasonably homogeneous form, resulting in a well-resolved spectrum of an apparently well-vascularized tumor with neutral pH (Fig. 5a). A single interferon treatment (50000 units in 0.1 ml administered s.c.) had little effect on the metabolic state of this tumor (Fig. 5b, c).

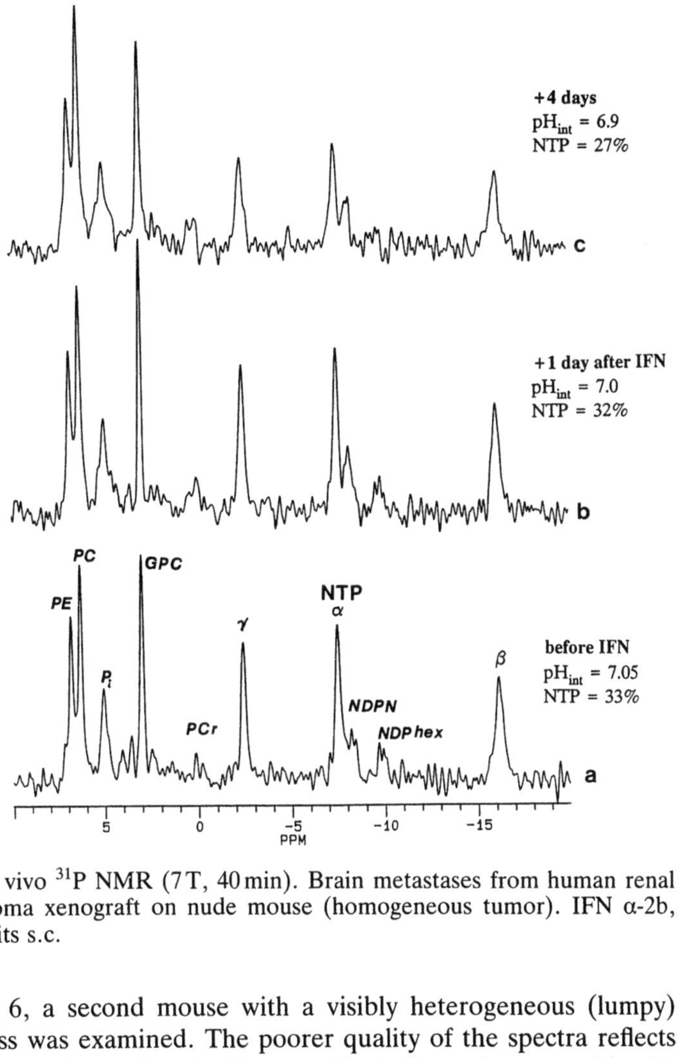

Fig. 5. In vivo ^{31}P NMR (7 T, 40 min). Brain metastases from human renal cell carcinoma xenograft on nude mouse (homogeneous tumor). IFN α-2b, 5×10^4 units s.c.

In Fig. 6, a second mouse with a visibly heterogeneous (lumpy) tumor mass was examined. The poorer quality of the spectra reflects this heterogeneity, and a significant acidosis (hypoxia, necrosis) with increasing depth into the tumor could be seen based on the position of the phosphate resonance. Figure 7 shows the result of treating this tumor with interferon, and in this case a dramatic degradation of NTP and phosphoesters and liberation of P_i could be seen. The pH determined from the P_i signal increased gradually from 6.6 to 6.9 and became more uniform. This single treatment was not completely successful, however, and a gradual recovery of GPC and NTP levels could be detected after 6 days.

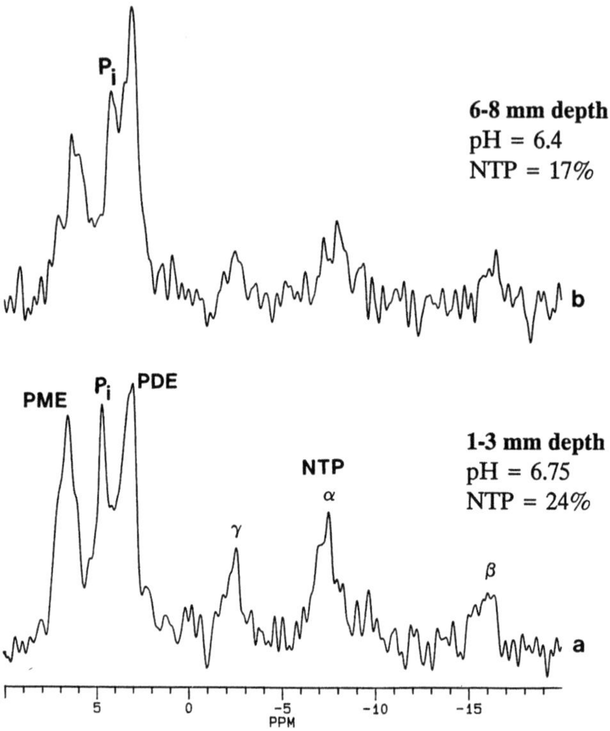

Fig. 6. In vivo ^{31}P NMR (7T, 40 min). Brain metastasis from human renal cell carcinoma xenograft on nude mouse (Large, heterogeneous, hypoxic tumor)

Conclusions and Prospects

Our initial in vitro NMR experiments with RCC have shown that:

- Human RCC cultures can be maintained in BMG and give high quality ^{31}P NMR spectra (ca. 5×10^7 cells).
- Compared with other tumor lines the RCC line examined exhibited high levels of PE, GPC, and GPE, but low PC, even though only choline and not ethanolamine was present in the medium.
- Response to hyperthermia at 42.4°C was minor.
- Response to interferon-α was rapid; within 1 h there was a dramatic loss of PE, PCr, and nucleotides, but not a complete killing of cells.

Initial in vivo experiments with xenografts from a brain metastasis from an RCC patient have shown that:

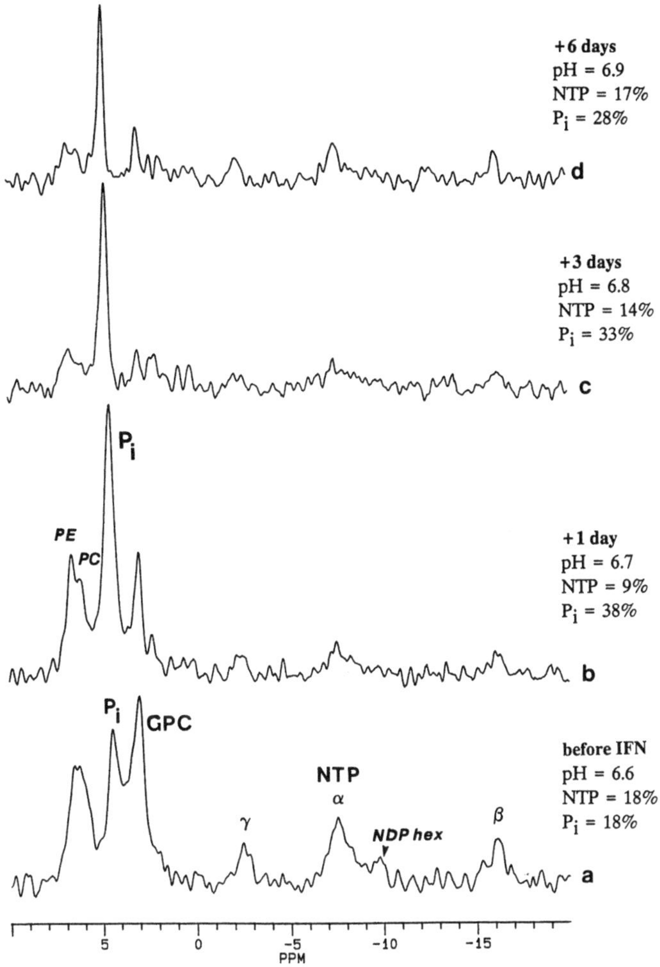

Fig. 7. In vivo ^{31}P NMR (7T, 40 min). Brain metastasis from human renal cell carcinoma xenograft on nude mouse (hypoxic tumor). IFN α-2b 5 × 10^4 units s.c.

- A small (1.5 cm) homogeneous tumor showed neutral pH, high nucleotide levels and no response to a single dose of interferon-α (50 000 units).
- A large (2.5 cm) heterogeneous and hypoxic tumor had a mean pH of ca. 6.6–6.7 and significantly lower nucleotide levels; the response to interferon-α was strong; nucleotides and phosphoesters degraded to P_i, which showed a homogeneous pH of 6.9 (perhaps extracellular?); after 6 days resynthesis of NTP was evident.

A wide range of further experiments can be envisaged:

- Compare various RCC lines with one another; correlate metabolic profiles with type and grading.
- Compare the same RCC line in culture and in vivo.
- Investigate in vitro and in vivo treatments with IFN and TNF alone and combined (does TNF induce hypoxia in vivo?).
- Investigate other cytokine or immunotherapies.
- Investigate other metabolites and pathways using ^{1}H (lactate production), ^{13}C (glycogen storage) and ^{19}F NMR (fluoropyrimidine chemotherapy).

References

Daly PF, Lyon RC, Straka EJ, Cohen JS (1988) ^{31}P NMR spectroscopy of human cancer cells proliferating in a basement membrane gel. FASEB J 2: 2596–2604

Daly PF, Cohen JS (1989) Magnetic resonance spectroscopy of tumors and potential in-vivo clinical applications: a review. Cancer Res 49: 770–779

Daly PF, Zugmaier G, Sandler D, Carpen M, Myers CE, Cohen JS (1990) Regulation of the cytidine phospholipid pathways in human cancer cells and effects of 1-β-D-arabinofuranosylcytosine: a non-invasive ^{31}P NMR study. Cancer Res 50: 552–557

Hull EW, Kuesel AC, Graschew G, Lorenz W, Thielmann HW (1990) High-field ^{21}P NMR studies of several human tumor cell lines. Comparisons in basement membrane gel culture and in solid tumors. Abstracts: Soc Magn Reson Med 9: 845

Kuesel AC, Graschew G, Hull WE, Lorenz W, Thielmann HW (1990) ^{31}P NMR studies of cultured human cells. Influence of pH on phospholipid metabolite levels and the detection of cytidine 5′-diphosphate choline. NMR in Biomed 3: 78–89

Neeman M, Rushkin E, Kadouri A, Degani H (1988) Adaptation of culture methods for NMR studies of anchorage-dependent cells. Magn Reson Med 7: 236–242

Neeman M, Degani H (1989) Metabolic studies of estrogen- and tamoxifen-treated human breast cancer cells by NMR spectroscopy. Cancer Res 49: 589–594

Neeman M, Degani H (1989) Early estrogen-induced metabolic changes and their inhibition by actinomycin D and cycloheximide in human breast cancer cells: ^{31}P and ^{13}C NMR studies. Proc Natl Acad Sci USA 86: 5585–5589

Steen RG (1989) Response of solid tumors to chemotherapy monitored by in-vivo ^{31}P nuclear magnetic resonance spectroscopy: a review. Cancer Res 49: 4075–4085

Conservative Surgery of Renal Tumors: Operative Technique, Complications, Results, DNA Cytometry

F. Steinbach[1], M. Stöckle[1], J.W. Thüroff[2], S. Störkel[3], S.W. Melchior[1], S.C. Müller[1], and R. Hohenfellner[1]

Introduction

Until now radical nephrectomy has been regarded as the standard therapy for nonmetastasized renal cell carcinoma. This operation has been accepted because of the theoretical advantage of a more complete resection. A parenchyma-sparing operation was only performed in patients in whom radical nephrectomy would result in renal failure requiring hemodialysis (imperative indication), such as patients with single kidney, bilateral tumors, dysfunctional contralateral kidney, or chronic renal failure. However, the widely used partial nephrectomy in these instances may in certain cases result in insufficient residual renal parenchyma. Simple enucleation of the tumor with a small surrounding margin of normal renal tissue is an alternative technique to this approach. The surprisingly good prognosis of patients who were treated by enucleation in the imperative group [1] has encouraged us over the past 9 years to perform parenchyma-sparing operations also in patients with small peripheral tumors and normal contralateral kidneys (elective indication). Moreover, these small and mostly asymptomatic kidney tumors which only a few years ago were rarely diagnosed, are being detected more frequently by ultrasound. Thus, the incidence of asymptomatic renal tumors increased from 10% in 1978 to 70% in 1989, while the classic symptoms of flank pain, hematuria and palpable mass were found in less than 10% of the cases. In this chapter we present the operative technique, compli-

[1] Urologische Klink and Poliklinik, Langenbeckstr. 1, W-6500 Mainz, FRG
[2] Urologische Klinik in Klinikum Barmen, Heusnerstr. 40, W-5600 Wuppertal 2, FRG
[3] Institut für Pathologie der Universität, Langenbeckstr. 1, W-6500 Mainz, FRG

G. Staehler S. Pomer (Eds.)
Basic and Clinical Research on Renal Cell Carcinoma

cations, patient outcome, and preliminary results of image analysis DNA cytometry.

Patients and Methods

Patients

Between 1969 and 1989 conservative surgery of kidney tumors was performed in 123 patients. Conservative surgery was imperative for 49 of the patients (18 female, 31 male) aged 38 to 77 years (average age 59 years). A total of 23 patients had metachronous or synchronous bilateral tumors, 12 patients had a single kidney, 9 patients a pathology of the contralateral kidney and 5 patients a chronic renal failure. In three cases metastases were present at the time of operation. In the imperative group, 17 tumors were diagnosed incidentally, 14 were linked with unspecific systems, and 18 with specific symptoms. Elective parenchyma-sparing surgery was performed on 74 patients (25 female, 49 male) aged 31 to 74 years (average age 55 years). Of these patients, 55 (74%) were asymptomatic; the tumor was discovered incidentally during an ultrasound examination. Unspecific symptoms (loss of weight and energy, increased blood sedimentation rate) was found in ten patients; specific urological symptoms (flank pain, hematuria, urinary tract infection) were present in nine patients.

Tumor Material for DNA Cytometry

Paraffin-embedded tumor tissue from 57 enucleated renal tumors was available for image analysis DNA cytometry. In 20 of these patients the indication for conservative surgery was imperative; the other 37 patients had an elective enucleation of their renal tumors. Forty nine of the enucleated tumors were renal cell carcinomas, six patients had an oncocytoma, one patient had an angiomyolipoma, and one a renal cell adenoma.

Surgical Technique

The kidney is exposed by a supracostal incision in the tenth or eleventh intercostal space. After opening Gerota's fascia, the kidney is freed from the surrounding fatty tissue. Only the tissue lying directly on the surface of the tumor is left and removed later along with the tumor. If the tumor is large or located in an unfavorable position (central location), the renal artery and vein are exposed and looped to facilitate clamping in an emergency situation. A sharp incision is made 3 to 5 mm from the tumor. Blunt enucleation is facilitated by the pseudocapsule surrounding most tumors. The smaller vessels between the renal parenchyma and the tumor are coagulated; the larger ones are ligated. Careful attention must by paid during enucleation in the deepest part of the tumor bed, as there is a danger of tearing the main vessels or damaging the underlying renal calyces. The completeness of enucleation is proved by multiple frozen sections from the tumor bed or the kidney tissue surrounding the enucleated tumor. In addition, the cavity is denaturated by an infrared coagulator. In small defects, suture of the capsula fibrosa is sufficient; larger defects are filled with surrounding fatty tissue. Regional lymphadenectomy is not routinely performed.

Image Analysis DNA Cytometry

A new type of the LEYTAS II system [7] (the "Modular Image Analysis Computer," MIAC, LEITZ Company, Wetzlar, Germany) was used for the automated analysis of the 4-acetamide-4′-isothiocyano-2,2′-disulfostilbene (SITS) stained smear preparations using the Feulgen method. This system automatically screens smear preparations of the tumors for cells of interest. The aim of this technique is to obtain DNA histograms which are selectively based on the tumor cell population. The majority of nontumorous cells, such as inflammatory or mesenchymal cells, are excluded on the basis of their different morphology.

The system uses an Autoplan microscope in combination with a × 40 objective, analyzing 512 × 512 µm fields at pixel separation of 1 µm. Simultaneous analysis of 128 × 128 µm fields at a pixel separation of 0.25 µm is accomplished by separating the light beam into two different channels for high and low magnification after passage through the objective. These two light channels are projected to two TV cameras. For screening of the slide, automatic focusing of the cells, and measurement of the DNA content of the cells of interest, the slide is moved in three dimensions by three different computer-controlled motors. Simultaneous screening of the slide at low magnification and cell analysis at high magnification has significantly accelerated the process. Within 20 min the screening and analysis of

300 nuclei can be performed if the preparation does not contain too many artifacts. The connection of the televized microscopic image to the MIAC, which utilizes a Motorola 68000 microprocessor, facilitates a rapid image analysis. The principles of mathematic morphology, as developed by Meyer [4], are the basis for a rapid image analysis. The microscopic image is digitized within 20 ms, allowing simultaneous analysis of all objects, and all that are of interest are automatically moved to the center of the image where cytophotometrical measurement is performed.

Simultaneously the high magnification image of the nucleus is scanned by an artifact rejection program. Automated image analysis is stopped when 320 cells have been counted or when all microscope fields have been screened. Pictures of all analyzed cells were stored in a memory buffer and subsequently controlled by the operator to exclude overlooked artifacts. In doubtful cases a computer command allowed immediate visualization of the object of interest on the microscope. The mathematical morphological criteria used for cells selection can be adapted for tumor types of different morphology, ensuring that not only artifacts such as a dirt or cell doublets, but also nontumorous cells like lymphocytes, granulocytes or spindle-shaped mesenchymal cells, can be excluded from the analysis. This results in DNA histograms which are selectively based on tumor cells and nontumorous epithelial cells surrounding the tumor, which represent a good internal diploid standard.

Preparation of Feulgen-Stained Tumor Cell Smears

Quantitative measurement of DNA content requires the analysis of intact nuclei. For this reason cytological smear preparations are more easily analyzed than histological sections, which unavoidably contain many overlapping and nonintact nuclei. A modified Hedley technique was used to prepare a single cell suspension from 50 μm sections of the tumors. The suspension was centrifuged on polyethylene-coated slides, which achieved equal distribution and separation of the nuclei in an identical focus plane, facilitating automated analysis of the smears.

Acriflavine and Sits Staining by the Feulgen Method

The smear preparations were fixed with carbowax (1% polyethyleneglycol in 50% ethanol), air-dried, and stained automatically by programmable staining machines (Shandon Company). In addition, a smear preparation of normal renal tissue was stained with every series as an exact diploid standard. Acriflavine–Feulgen binds quantitatively to DNA and allows selective absorption cytophotometry at 466 nm wave length. UV fluorescense demonstrates the nucleoli and cellular proteins, facilitating cytomorphological analysis of the smear preparations.

Follow-up

During the first postoperative year a control check-up (physical examination, blood and urine tests, chest X-ray, kidney and liver sonography) was performed every 3 months, and thereafter every 6 months. If sonography revealed no pathological findings, a computed tomography was done yearly.

Results

Histology

Histological classification was carried out according to the classification scheme described by Thoenes et al. [10]. In the imperative group, 21 grade I renal cell carcinomas (RCCs) were found; 17 were of grade II and 7 grade III. In 4 cases the histology revealed an oncocytoma. The average tumor size was 5.2 cm and varied from 2 to 11 cm. In the elective group, 13 benign lesions were found (1 adenoma, 1 fibroma, 1 angiomyolipoma, 1 leiomyoma, 1 hemorrhagic cyst, and 8 oncocytomas). In 34 cases the RCC was diagnosed as grade I, in 23 grade II and in 4 patients grade III. Tumor size varied from 1 to 7 cm (mean 3.2 cm).

Imperative Group

Follow-up in the imperative group ranged from 5 months to 17.3 years, with an average length of 4.5 years. In this group, 36 of 49 patients are alive with no evidence of disease. In three of the six patients who died of tumor progression, the operation had been only palliative as metastases were already present. These operations were performed because selective embolization technique to control the bleeding complications was not yet available. In two patients a second tumor, not located in the original tumor bed, occurred 1 and 5 years postoperatively. Both were treated successfully with further enucleation. One of these patients remained tumor free for 63 months after his second operation. The other patient developed lung metastases which were treated successfully with immunization therapy. One further patient died due to postoperative bleeding with consecutive hypovolemic shock. Four patients died of diseases unrelated to the tumor. In two cases no follow-up data are available. Postoperative serum-creatinine levels remained unchanged, except in one patient with chronic renal failure in whom the creatinine increased from 2.5 to 4.3 mg/dl after enucleation of a tumor 11 cm in diameter.

Elective Group

Follow-up in the elective group ranged from 5 months to 8.3 years, with a mean follow-up period of 3.3 years. Of the 74 patients, 68 are alive with no evidence of disease. In one patient whose preoperative cranial CT scan was normal in spite of neurological symptoms, a brain metastasis was diagnosed and removed 2 years after enucleation. The patient died of further distant metastases without evidence of a local tumor recurrence. In two patients a second renal tumor occurred 4 and 5 years after the first enucleation, one tumor in the original tumor bed, and the other at a different location in the kidney. Both were treated successfully, one by a second enucleation, and one by radical nephrectomy. The patients are alive without evidence of tumor progression. One patient was lost to follow-up; three died due to diseases unrelated to the tumor. None of the patients with a benign lesion developed a further tumor. Postoperative serum creatinine remained stable in all patients except one, who showed an increase of 0.5 mg/dl.

Image Analysis DNA Cytometry

Three main types of renal tumors could be distinguished from one another on the basis of the DNA histogram: diploid tumors (n = 32); (Fig. 1a), tetraploid tumors (n = 5); (Fig. 1b), and aneuploid tumors (n = 20); (Fig. 1c). Within the group of aneuploid tumors, several subtypes could be found: hyperdiploid tumors (n = 8) which had a stem cell line with DNA content between 2 and 2.5 C and showed a closed correlation with the tumor type histologically classified as

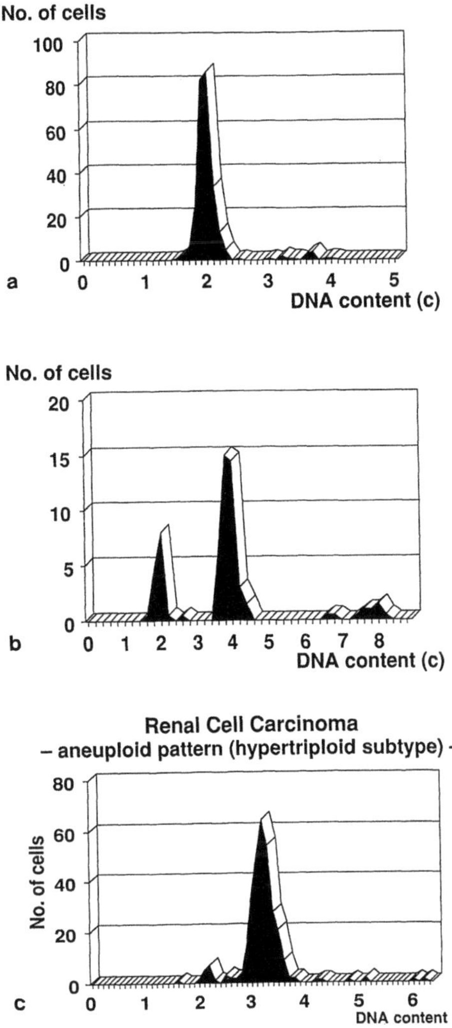

Fig. 1. **a** Diploid tumor ($n = 32$). The stem-cell line at 2c shows the same DNA content as nontumorous epithelial renal cells which have been analysed as diploid standard. **b** Diploid-tetraploid tumor ($n = 6$). Octoploid cells can be documented in addition to the diploid and tetraploid ones which also characterize the diploid tumor. **c** Hypertriploid tumor ($n = 2$); these two patients were the only one who died of their tumor. The absence of a diploid peak indicates that the nontumorous cell elements can efficiently be eliminated by the image analysis system

papillary chromophil. A hypertriploid tumor was found in two patients and is characterized by a stem cell line between 3 and 4C (Fig. 1c). A hypertetraploid stem cell line with more than 4C DNA content was found in two patients. Eight tumors showed a combination of diploid and hypertriploid cells. Of the 49 renal cell carcinomas, 26 were diploid, five tetraploid, eight hyperdiploid, two hypertriploid, one hypertetraploid and seven were diploid/hypertriploid. Of the six oncocytomas the DNA histograms revealed four diploid, one diploid/hypertriploid and one having a hypertetraploid pattern. The angiomyolipoma as well as the renal cell adenoma showed a diploid DNA histogram.

Correlation of the DNA Histogram with the Clinical Course of the Patients

The two patients with a pure hypertriploid tumor died of distant metastases without local recurrence. In both cases the survival times were 3 years. One of the patients had an imperative and one an elective indication for conservative resection of the renal tumor. One female patient with a diploid-hypertriploid tumor underwent a second tumor resection several years after the first enucleation because of a heterotopic tumor recurrence in her solitary kidney. After 3 more years the CT scan revealed two small lesions for which malignancy diagnosis was uncertain as well as lung metastases. Complete remission of the lung metastases as well as stable disease of the kidney lesions was achieved by the use of a specific vaccination therapy using autologous tumor cells. All other patients are alive without evidence of disease.

Operative Complications

Operative complications within the imperative and elective groups are as follows:

1. Imperative group
   - One postoperative hemorrhage resulting in hypovolemic shock and subsequent death
   - One injury of the spleen with secondary splenectomy
   - One urine skin fistula and one urinoma, which were treated by ureteral catheterization
   - Two pulmonary embolisms without further complications

2. Elective group
   - One septic pyelonephritis with secondary nephrectomy
   - One retroperitoneal urinoma and one hematoma, which were treated conservatively
   - One pulmonary embolism without further complications

Discussion

Conservative surgery of renal tumors has been performed in our department since 1969, initially only in patients with an imperative indication [1]. The results in this group have demonstrated the sufficiency of these techniques to preserve the renal function and encouraged us in the early 1980s to extend the indication for conservative surgery to small, peripherally located tumors with healthy contralateral kidneys (elective indication). This concept has been facilitated by the increasingly early identification of these mostly asymptomatic tumors as a result of modern diagnostic procedures, especially sonography and CT. These tumors have often been so small that radical nephrectomy seemed not to be justified, even in the presence of a healthy contralateral kidney. The results in this group seem to confirm the strategy of conservative surgery of renal tumors with an elective indication. They are based on an average follow-up period of 3.3 years; in 20 patients with a RCC the follow-up time of no evidence of disease is about 5 years. In the one patient in this group who developed metastases, it can be assumed that occult metastases were already present preoperatively. According to our study a more conservative approach to small, peripherally located tumors is confirmed in the recent literature [5, 6]. In an Austrian Multicenter Study including 52 patients with an elective indication for conservative surgery the survival rate was comparable to results after radical nephrectomy in cases of low tumor stage [6]. However, the RCC is an unpredictable tumor that has been known to recur as late as 13 years after the first operation, and it may remain stable for a period of 35 years when untreated, so all results should be cautiously interpreted. The low operative complication rate and the unpredictability of whether small renal lesions are malignant are further reasons for elective enucleation of renal tumors. Although the specificity of CT scan in the diagnosis of small renal tumors is 90%, the differentiation of oncocytomas, adenomas and hemorrhagic cyst is difficult. In our patients all oncocytomas and two of the other five benign tumors had been assumed preoperatively to be RCCs. In these cases radical nephrectomy would have been an unacceptable overtreatment. Final evaluation of magnetic resonance imaging (MRI) in the diagnosis of renal tumors cannot be given at this time. Furthermore, a biopsy of renal tumors carries the risk of bleeding and spilling of tumor cells, and even negative results at cytological examination does not rule out a malignant tumor. A serious argument for organ-preserving surgery is the risk of developing a tumor in the contralateral kidney after radical nephrectomy, which occurs in 1.8% to 3.8% of patients. Of our own patients, 23 presented with bilateral tumors, either synchronously or metachronously, in one case 15 years after the first operation. The major concern about organ-preserving surgery for RCC in patients with a normal contralateral kidney is the risk of multifocality, which has an incidence of 0.5% to 5% in the literature [8]. Excluded from this argumentation are patients with von Hippel-Lindau's disease, of whom 75% have bilateral tumors, and in whom multiple recurrent lesions are common. An optimal parenchyma-sparing operation, like enucleation, is the treatment of choice in these cases. Three of our patients developed further kidney tumors which could be traced to a multifocal RCC. The risk of missing a multifocal tumor in the follow-up period could be reduced significantly by the improvement of diagnostic techniques (ultrasound, CT scan). Furthermore, it is important to determine whether multifocality is a unilateral or bilateral disease. Our clinical results suggested that partial nephrectomy is not superior to the method of tumor enucleation presented here, although Marshall et al. [3] have reported residual tumor in kidneys after ex vivo enucleations in radical nephrectomy specimens. These findings are not confirmed in the series of Morgan and Zincke [5], who found no significant difference in outcome between enucleation and partial nephrectomy. Enucleation is the most widely accepted surgical procedure for tumors throughout the kidney, and central lesions, and in patients with von Hippel-Lindau's disease. Enucleation is most controversial when it concerns the polar located tumor, in which a partial nephrectomy is most easily performed. We try to minimize the risk of incomplete tumor enucleation by using the following operative procedures: tumor enucleation at a distance 3–5 mm from the tumor, multiple frozen sections of the tumor bed, and infrared coagulation of the cavity. The completely freed kidney is inspected and palpated carefully to detect further tumor lesions.

The results of automated image analysis DNA cytometry of enucleated renal tumors indicate that the term renal cell carcinoma includes a heterogeneous variety of different tumors rather than a homogeneous disease entity [9]. Histological analysis also differentiates a broad variety of RCCs. DNA cytometric findings and histological results, however, showed a close correlation only between the papillary-clear cell type and the hyperdiploid type. The tetraploid renal tumor type (Fig. 1b) could be a phenomenon of polyploidy, which is characterized by a combination of diploid, tetraploid and octoploid tumor cells. Such tetraploid cells are characterized by their ability to divide into two diploid cells, whereas aneuploidy is an irreversible phenomenon. Only the two patients with a pure hypertriploid tumor have died of tumor progression, indicating a close correlation between the prognosis and DNA histogram of the tumor. DNA analysis of bladder cancer specimens also revealed that hypertriploid tumors have the poorest prognosis. However, further analysis of a larger series of patients with advanced RCC is necessary to evaluate the prognostic relevance and potential therapeutic consequences of the DNA histograms. Ljungberg et al. [2] made the statement, based on flow cytometric analysis of metastasized RCCs, that patients with "diploid or peridiploid" tumors, in contrast to patients with aneuploid tumors, benefited from aggressive surgical therapy, including resection of metastases. A minority of tumors respond impressively to immunologic therapeutic modalities. It remains to be seen whether automated image analysis DNA cytometry will provide criteria which will predict the response to such treatment modalities and, therefore, allow more individual therapeutic planning. The hyperdiploid-aneuploid tumor type described by Stöckle et al. [9] has not been previously characterized in the literature. It was probably subsumed under the term "diploid and peridiploid" tumors [2], because the technology used was not sufficiently accurate to distinguish these two types of tumors. As compared to DNA flow cytometry [7], automated image analysis DNA cytometry, utilizing programmable morphological selection criteria, allows the selective analysis of the tumor cells, and the majority of nontumor cells can be excluded from the measurement. Furthermore, it provides an easy and repeatable access for the cytological analysis of tumor cell smears. The rapid development in hardware and software has reduced the time necessary for DNA cytometry and the use of image analysis. This allows a routine use of the method in our laboratory.

It is highly important to inform the patients in advance of the operative technique and related risks of elective tumor enucleation as well as the necessity of close follow-up controls. Patients with a low compliance should be excluded from an elective conservative surgery of RCCs.

References

1. Bazeed MA, Schärfe T, Becht E, Jurincic C, Alken P, Thüroff JW (1986) Conservative surgery of renal cell carcinoma. Eur Urol 12: 238–243
2. Ljungberg B, Stenling R, Roos G (1986) Prognostic value of deoxyribonucleid acid content in metastatic renal cell carcinoma. J Urol 136: 801–804
3. Marshall FF, Taxy JB, Fishman EK, Chang R (1986) The feasibility of surgical enucleation for renal cell carcinoma. J Urol 135: 231
4. Meyer F (1979) Interative image transformation for an automatic screening of cervical smears. J Histochem Cytochem 27: 128–135
5. Morgan WR, Zincke H (1990) Progression and survival after renal-conserving surgery for renal cell carcinoma: Experience in 104 patients and extended follow-up. J Urol 144: 852
6. Petritsch PH, Rauchenwald M, Zechner O, et al. (1990) Results after organ-preserving surgery for renal cell carcinoma. An Austrian multicenter study. Eur Urol 18: 84
7. Ploem JS, van Driel-Kulker AMJ, Verwoerd NP (1987) LEYTAS a cytology screening system using the new modular image analysis computer (MIAC) from Leitz. In: Burger Z, Ploem JS, Goerttler H (eds) Clinical cytometry and histometry. Academic Press, London, pp 24–35
8. Sparwasser C, Bach D, Sparwasser H, Altwein JE (1984) Das bilaterale Hypernephrom. Akt Urol 15: 312
9. Stöckle M, Störkel S, Miehlke R, Steinbach F, Galler E, Riedmiller H, Hohenfellner R (1990) Charakterisierung konservativ operierter Nierentumoren mit der automatisierten DNS-Bildzytometrie. Akt Urol 21: 173
10. Thoenes W, Störkel S, Rumpelt HJ (1986) Histopathology and classification of renal cell tumors (adenomas, oncocytomas and carcinomas). The basic cytological and histopathological elements and their use for diagnostics. Pathol Pract 181: 125–143

Clinical Relevance of Proliferation Rates in Renal Cell Carcinoma

W. de Riese[1], E.P. Allhoff[1], C.G. Stief[1], R. Schlick[1], P. Anton[1], and U. Jonas[1]

Flemming (1882) and Waldeyer (1888) were the first to describe the histomorphological conception of cell division, mitosis and cell proliferation in human malignancies [5]. In different malignant tumors, pathologists found a correlation between mitosis rate determined in histological specimens and the clinical course of patients with malignancies. Mitosis, however, plays only a small part in the active cell cycle and is therefore only an indirect parameter of the proliferative pattern of the tissue. A long time passed before direct detection of tumor-specific proliferation rates (PRs) was possible. Through autoradiographic studies using the thymidine incorporation assay direct measurement of the portion of DNA synthesizing cells became available. In 1979, H.M. Rabes and his coworkers presented a clinical report of PR in renal cell carcinoma (RCC) using this technique [10]. They found a correlation between PR and recurrence rate in a series of ten patients. The main disadvantages of the thymidine incorporation technique are (a) extracorporal organ perfusion (ex vivo) after tumor nephrectomy and (b) radioactivity; therefore, it is not a practicable technique for routine diagnosis.

The preparation of monoclonal antibodies was a relevant step towards solving these problems. In 1983 Gerdes and his coworkers isolated and characterized a human nuclear antigen (termed Ki-67) present only in DNA synthesizing cells [2]. This characteristic is present in both normal and malignant cells, but is absent in resting cells, as illustrated schematically for the different parts of the cell cycle in Fig. 1 [4]. By using frozen sections and the afore-mentioned immunohistochemical staining technique, in vivo proliferation rates

[1] Medizinische Hochschule Hannover, Urologische Klinik, Konstanty-Gutschow Str. 8, W-3000 Hannover 61, FRG

G. Staehler S. Pomer (Eds.)
Basic and Clinical Research on Renal Cell Carcinoma

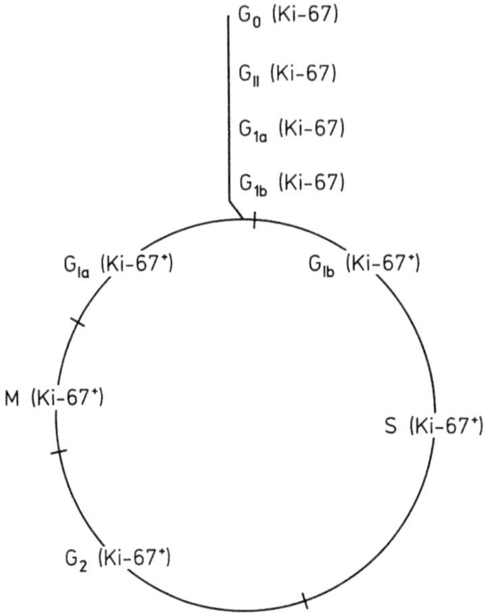

Fig. 1. Occurrence of the cell proliferation-associated nuclear antigen (Ki-67) in the different phases of cell cycle. (According to Gerdes et al. [4])

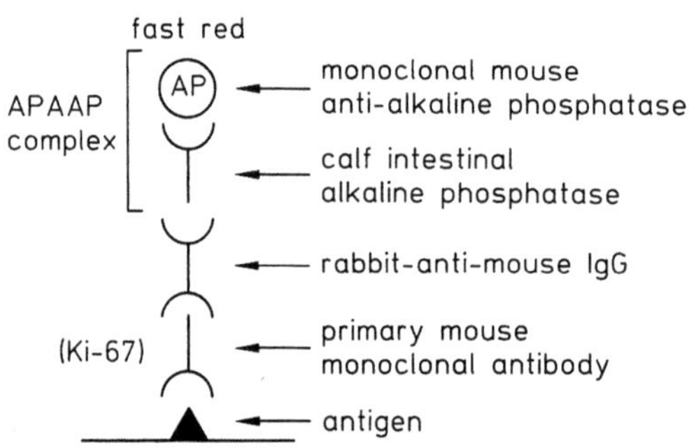

Fig. 2. Schematic representation of the immunohistochemical (Ki-67) staining technique using the 'APAAP complex'. (According to Cordell et al. [1]).

of normal and malignant tissue can now be directly determined [3] (Fig. 2).

As illustrated in Fig. 3, the time of the collection of the specimen is important for the correct determination of the individual PR. It can be seen that, 3.5 h after tumor nephrectomy, PR is only approxi-

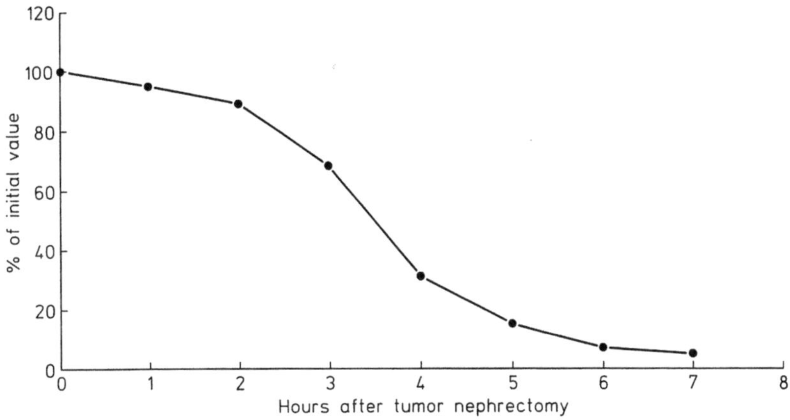

Fig. 3. Impact of the time of the specimen collection on PR (mean values of 10 different RCC tumors)

mately half of the initial PR. These data correlate with the in vitro success rates of tumor cells, depending on the time of cell preparation [6, 12]. The determination of the percentage of Ki-67 positive cells was performed as described by Gerdes [3]. In order to exclude sampling error it is necessary to take several samples of solid tumor tissue, depending on the individual tumor size (Table 1). The highest PR of all analyzed specimens is representative of the entire tumor.

In correlation with the data published by Rabes [10], higher PRs were always measured in the peripheral zones of the tumors rather than in the central zones. This is obviously nutrition related due to a better blood circulation in the peripheral areas. Furthermore, necrosis and cysts develop first in the central zones of tumors, as has often been macroscopically observed.

Table 1. Representative sampling for measurement of PR[a] depends on tumor size

Size of tumor	Number of specimens	
	Peripheral	Central
< 3 cm	2	1
3–6 cm	4	2
> 6 cm	6	2

PR, proliferation rates
[a] PR of peripheral tumors are greater than that of central tumors.

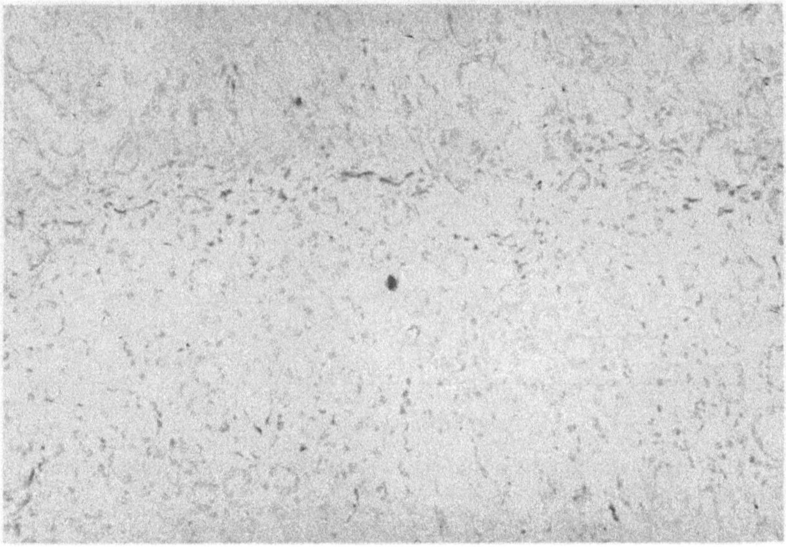

Fig. 4. Normal renal tissue, immunohistochemical staining with the mab Ki-67, positive cells stained dark. (Original magnification × 80)

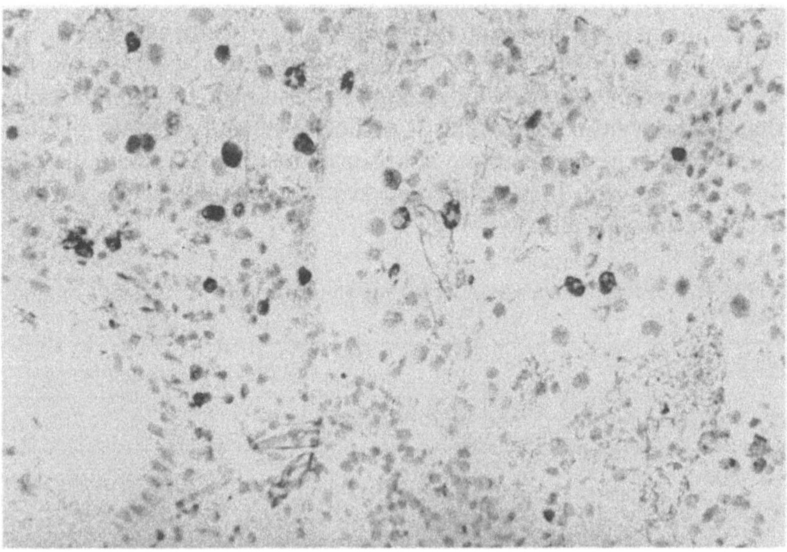

Fig. 5. High grade (G 3), low differentiated RCC, Ki 67 staining technique, PR = 18%. (Original magnification × 120)

Table 2. Correlation of tumor stage (pT) and grade (G) with proliferation rates in 110 patients[a] with renal cell carcinoma

	Proliferation rates		
	0%–4% (n)	>4%–9% (n)	>9% (n)
pT 1–2	31	24	16 (N.S.)
pT 3	10	17	12 (N.S.)
G 1	25 (74%)*	7	2
G 2	24	12	14
G 3	3	8	15 (58%)*

* $p < 0.05$
[a] Data are from 1986–1990 in patients with T1-3, No, Mo tumors.

From 1986 until 1990, the PRs of 110 RCC patients were immunohistochemically measured by the Ki-67 assay, as described above. According to histology and imaging techniqes these patients were without evidence of metastatic disease at the time of tumor nephrectomy. Whereas normal renal tissue has a PR of less than 1% (Fig. 4), malignant renal tissue exhibits PRs ranging from 1% to 18% (Fig. 5). Table 2 gives an overview of PR, histological tumor staging (pT) and grading (G) of the 110 investigated cases. The classification of all RCCs was performed according to the actual TNM system of the

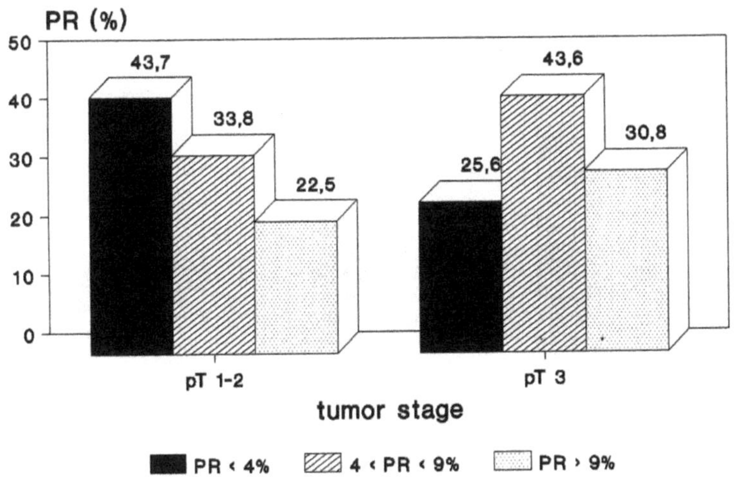

Fig. 6. Distribution of proliferation rates (PR) related to tumor stage (pT)

UICC [7]. There is no correlation between individual PR and tumor stage (pT) (Fig. 6). In contrast to these findings a strong correlation between PR and tumor grade (G) is observed (Fig. 7). In early stages (pT1–2) fivefold varying PRs are measured. From individual PRs the individual tumor stage cannot be concluded, because tumor stage is a function of cell proliferation and time, which is not determinable at time of diagnosis. We observed large tumors with low PRs and small tumors (less than 3 cm in diameter) with PRs above 9%. These data confirm clinical findings without tumor progression observed over a long time period in RCC patients who were not operated on for different reasons [8, 11].

Fifteen (16.3%) of the 110 patients of this ongoing study have developed recurring tumors (mean follow-up: 2.8 years). Eleven patients with tumor recurrence during the follow-up period exhibited PRs above 9% at the time of tumor nephrectomy; the remaining four patients showed PRs ranging from 4% to 9%. Three patients with early tumor stages (pT1–2) and recurrence had PRs above 9%. These data correspond to the results of PRs in breast cancer presented by Lelle et al. (1987) [9]: a positive correlation between histological grading, recurrence rate and PRs was observed.

In conclusion, the immunohistochemical determination of the tumor-specific PR using the monoclonal antibody Ki-67 is a practicable, reliable and reproducible method complementary to conventional tumor staging and grading. The measurement of the individual

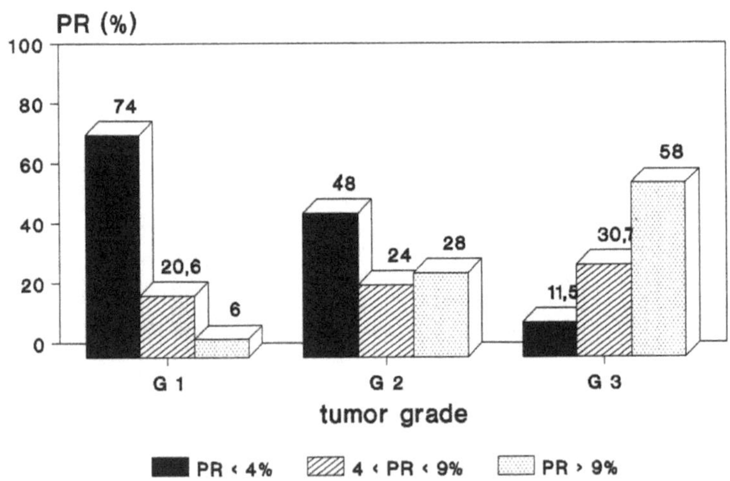

Fig. 7. Distribution of proliferation rates (PR) related to tumor grade (G)

PRs is an additional diagnostic parameter intended to detect RCC patients at high risk, especially at the early stages when histological staging and grading might be identical.

References

1. Cordell JL, Falini B, Erber NW, et al. (1984) Immunoenzymatic labeling of monoclonal antibodies using immune complexes of alkaline phosphatase and monoclonal antialkaline phosphatase (APAAP complexes). J Histochem Cytochem 32: 219–229
2. Gerdes J, Schwab U, Lemke H, Stein H (1983) Production of a mouse monoclonal antibody reactive with a human nuclear antigen associated with cell proliferation. Int J Cancer 31: 13–20
3. Gerdes J, Dallenbach F, Lennert K (1984) Growth fractions in malignant non-Hodgkin's lymphomas (NHL) as determined in situ with the monoclonal antibody Ki-67. Hemat Oncol 2: 365–371
4. Gerdes J, Lemke H, Baisch H, Wacker HH, Schwab U, Stein H (1984) Cell cycle analysis of a cell proliferation-associated human nuclear antigen defined by the monoclonal antibody Ki-67. J Immunol 133: 1710–1715
5. Girod C (1986) Die Entwicklung der Kenntnisse von der Zelle. In: Toellner R (Hrsg) Illustrierte Geschichte der Medizin. Rabe, Stuttgart, S 1884–1893
6. Hanauske AR, Von Hoff DD (1985) Clinical correlations with the human tumor cloning assay. Cancer Invest 3: 541–551
7. Hermanek P, Sobin LH (1987) Classification of urological tumors. In: Hermanek P, Sobin LH (eds) TNM classification of malignant tumors, 4th edn. Springer, Berlin Heidelberg New York Tokyo, pp 137–139
8. De Kernion JB (1986) Renal Tumors. In: Walsh PC, Gittes RF, Permutter AD, Stamey TA (eds) Campbell's Urology, 5th edn., vol 2. Saunders, Philadelphia, pp 1297–1342
9. Lelle RJ, Heidenreich W, Stauch G, Gerdes J (1987) The correlation of growth fractions with histologic grading and lymph node status in human mammary carcinoma. Cancer 59: 83–88
10. Rabes HM, Carl P, Meister P, Rattenhuber U (1979) Analysis of proliferative compartments in renal adenocarcinoma: Cancer 44: 799–804
11. Schorn A, Marberger M (1984) Long-term survival of untreated bilateral renal cell carcinoma with supradiaphragmatic vena caval thrombus. J Urol 131: 108–109
12. Von Hoff DD (1987) In-vitro predictive testing. Int J Cell Cloning 5: 179–190

Chemotherapy of Renal Cell Carcinoma

Cytotoxic Chemotherapy Phase II Trials Between 1983 and 1990 for Advanced Renal Cell Carcinoma

A. Yagoda[1]

Introduction

Cytotoxic chemotherapy has been and continues to be a disappointing therapeutic modality for metastatic and recurrent renal cell carcinoma, as is evidenced by less than 5% to 15% of cases achieving significant tumor regression, that is, complete remission (CR) and partial (PR) remission [3, 4, 10]. While chemotherapy has become an integral component of multidisciplinary therapies for most solid tumors, the absence of even modest antitumor activity against advanced renal cell cancer has led to the continued need for further disease-oriented phase II studies to define efficacy. Additionally, without defined efficacy, presently available drugs have no role either adjuvantly or neoadjuvantly.

Analysis of results of pre-1983 phase II studies of cytotoxic agents for renal cell carcinoma revealed that, at best, most of them induced CR or PR in only 0%–10% of cases, a rate which may simply represent "background noise" [3, 4]. Furthermore, because of the absence of significant antitumor response with agents used singly, it has not been surprising that multidrug combination regimens have also proved ineffective. This chapter reviews new, mostly phase II, disease-oriented trials of investigational cytotoxic drugs, as well as newer dosage schedules of older agents, evaluated between 1983 and 1990. (Only references not included in my earlier paper [10] are listed.)

Disease-oriented phase II studies, which are efficacy trials, require bidimensionally measurable parameters in order to define a clear

[1] Columbia Presbyterian Medical Center, Atchley Pavilion, Room 735, 161 Fort Washington Avenue, New York, New York 10032-3784, USA

G. Staehler S. Pomer (Eds.)
Basic and Clinical Research on Renal Cell Carcinoma

end-point of response. Another frequent protocol entry requirement, particularly for renal cell carcinoma, is the absence of prior cytotoxic drugs, since recent findings have documented that renal tumors possess a "turned-on" expression of the multidrug resistant gene Mdr-1, and exposure to a prior agent can activate the gene, thereby hindering response to the agent being tested [1]. In fact, the presence of Mdr-1 may explain the consistent failure of cytotoxic agents against renal cancer, and, perhaps, any evidence of direct antitumor activity may be simply an indirect consequence of an effect on the immune system. Response criteria also are an important component of phase II trials. While CR and PR can be more readily defined, a major problem in evaluating reports of clinical trials in renal cell carcinoma involves stabilization of disease (STAB), a category which has been abused, particularly when used as evidence of an "objective" response. In some studies, STAB is defined as a change in tumor size from a decrease of less than 50% or less than 25% to an increase of less than 25% or even up to less than 50%. With the clinically recognized inaccuracies in the measurement of tumor size, by no stretch of the imagination can STAB be indicative of an "objective" and beneficial improvement; rather, it indicates the present inability to document slow progression of disease in sites which may be poorly evaluable because of the absence of sensitive biochemical and immunological diagnostic techniques to document tumor cell death. Moreover, the natural history of renal cell carcinoma suggests some element of heterogeneity, intermittent growth being coupled with spontaneous tumor regression in selected cases. While patients who achieve STAB should be continued on therapy until active tumor progression has been documented, this category should always be excluded from the reported "objective" response rate in order to avoid an exaggerated incidence of remission.

These silent statisticians – patient selection, tumor heterogeneity and definitions of response criteria – have influenced results of clinical trials in renal cell cancer, as well as in other solid tumors. Thus, only attainment of CR or PR status, coupled with their 95% confidence intervals (95% CI) for each percent response, is defined as an objective response (Table 1).

Results

The actions of many agents have still not been adequately elucidated and therefore, the various phase II drugs evaluated against renal cell

Table 1. New cytotoxic agents for renal cell carcinoma evaluated between 1983 and 1990. (Modified from Yagoda [10])

	Number	%CR/PR	95% CI
Mitotic Inhibitors:	*258*	*7*	*4–10*
Elliptinium	46	11	2–22
Taxol	18	0	0–16
Teniposide	95	4	0–18
Vinblastine, CI	99	8	3–13
Anthracyclines:	*243*	*3*	*2–4*
Epirubicin	39	0	0–7
Esorubicin	99	3	0–7
Idarubicin	19	0	0–15
Menogaril	70	4	0–9
THP ADM	16	6	0–18
Metal Agents:	*130*	*0*	*0–2*
Carboplatin	37	0	0–8
Gallium nitrate	35	0	0–8
Spirogermanium	62	0	0–4
Intercalating Drugs:	*413*	*2*	*1–3*
Amsacrine	140	1	0–3
Amonafide	27	0	0–11
Bisantrene	109	6	2–11
Mitoxantrone	137	1	0–3
Pyrimidines:	*231*	*15*	*4–26*
Deoxcytidine (DAC)	12	0	0–22
Fluroxidine (FUDR)	153	22	15–29
Sparfosic Acid (PALA)	66	3	0–7
Purines:	*154*	*1*	*0–3*
Acivicin (AT-125)	27	4	0–11
Alanosine	36	3	0–9
Aminothiadiazole	46	2	0–6
Fludarabine	45	0	0–6
Alkylating Agents:	*409*	*3*	*1–5*
Diaziquone (AZQ)	119	2	0–5
Cyclophosphamide + Interferon	21	5	0–14
Cyclophosphamide + Misonidazole	31	3	0–9
Ifosfamide	27	7	0–17
ICRF-187	40	0	0–6
Mitolactol	44	9	1–18
PCNU	79	1	0–3
Streptozotocin	18	6	0–17
Triepoxide (TGU)	30	0	0–10
Antifols:	*26*	*0*	*0–12*
10-Deaza-aminopterin	12	0	0–22
Trimetrexate	14	0	0–20

Table 1. *Continued*

	Number	%CR/PR	95% CI
Miscellaneous Agents:	*445*	*7*	*5–7*
Didemnin-B	44	2	0–6
Lonidamine	25	8	0–19
N-methylformamide	27	0	0–12
Mitoguazone	180	6	2–10
Cimetidine	25	8	3–19
Cimetidine + Coumarin	119	14	8–20
Cimetidine + Interferon	25	8	0–19

carcinoma have been grouped into the major classes of neoplastic agents; it must be recognized that some agents have been found to function somewhat differently than originally thought.

The accepted "standard" cytotoxic agent for renal cell carcinoma is the mitotic inhibitor, vinblastine sulfate, with a remission rate of 7% [4]. Recently, 5-day continuous infusions of vinblastine, which may be a more rational pharmacokinetic schedule, has been reevaluated in doses of 1.4–1.7 mg/m^2 day every 3–4 weeks [10]. Despite this, results are still disappointing, with only 8% (95% CI = 3%–13%) of 99 cases in four separate trials responding. Combinations of vinblastine and interferon have also been evaluated in both phase II and randomized phase III studies; such combinations have been found no more efficacious than either agent singly. Other new mitotic inhibitors, equally ineffective, are elliptinium (2-*n*-methyl-9-hydroxyellipticinium acetate, which is derived from the plant alkaloid ellipticine and may function as a DNA-intercalating agent) with a response rate of 11% (95% CI = 2%–20%) in 46 patients, and taxol (a drug which stabilizes microtubular depolymerization through binding to polymerized microtubules and is cross-resistant to vinblastine via the pleiotropic resistant gene) with no (95% CI = 0%–16%) remissions in 18 cases. Consequently, only 7% (95% CI = 4%–10%) of 258 cases given mitotic inhibitors obtained CR or PR.

Various anthracyclines continued to be evaluated including epirubicin (epidoxorubicin), esorubicin (4′ deoxydoxorubicin), idarubicin (demethoxydaunomycin), THP-ADM (4′-0-tetrahydro-pyranyl-adriamycin) and menogaril (an antibiotic derivative of nogalamycin which may have a different antitumor activity than that of doxorubicin evidenced by incomplete cross-resistance with the latter) [5, 10]. While one menogaril trial noted no activity in 14 cases [10], a cooperative group study in 56 cases described three (5%) remissions [7] for an overall rate of 4.3% (95% CI = 0%–9%). A remission rate of 3% (95% CI = 2%–4%) is noted in 243 cases given such anthracycline derivatives.

A new trial of carboplatin (a heavy metal which may function as an alkylating agent) in doses of 400 mg/m^2 has found no activity in 18 adequately treated cases [8]; this trial, combined with another study in 19 patients given either 450 mg/m^2 monthly or a dose calculated upon renal function [10], resulted in no remissions (95% CI = 0%–8%) in 37 cases. Gallium nitrate (another heavy metal agent, which induces hypocalcemia and also may function as an alkylating agent) was evaluated in two separate trials using either 700 mg/m^2 by bolus every 2 weeks or 100–200 mg/m^2 day for 7 days by continuous infusion. There was no (95% CI = 0%–8%) response in 35 patients. Spirogermanium (a compound containing germanium and a member of the azaspirane group) exhibited no (95% CI = 0%–4%) activity in 62 cases in doses of 80–120 mg/m^2. Metal-containing drugs, many of which function as alkylating agents, have not produced a single response (95% CI = 0%–2%) in 130 cases.

Intercalating agents evaluated are amsacrine, two anthracenedione derivatives – bisantrene and mitoxantrone – and amonafide, which may not function purely by intercalation. Responses have been observed in 1% (95% CI = 0%–3%) of 140, 6% (95% CI = 2%–11%) of 109, 1% (95% CI = 0%–3%) of 137, and 0% (95% CI = 0%–11%) of 27 cases, respectively. Overall, the rate is 2% (95% CI = 1%–3%) in 413 patients given such drugs [10].

Cyclophosphamide, 25 mg orally twice daily, combined with either recombinant alpha-2b-interferon or with misonidazole (a hypoxic cell radiosensitizer), induced one PR (95% CI = 0%–14%) in 21 cases (5%) and one PR (95% CI = 0%–9%) in 30 cases (3%), respectively. Other alkylating drug trials tried streptozotocin (a naturally occurring glucosamine nitrosurea), ifosfamide (a cyclophosphamide derivative), ICRF-187 (a derivative of razoxane), diaziquone, dibromodulcitol or mitolactol, 1, 2, 4-triglycidylurazol (a triepoxide), and PCNU (a new nitrosourea of the chlorethyl-piperidyl class). Overall, PR occurred in 3% (95% CI = 1%–5%) of 409 cases [10].

Two antifols evaluated, 10-deaza-aminopterin and trimetrexate, were inactive in trials of 12 and 14 evaluable patients, respectively (0%, 95% CI = 0%–12%) [10].

In 385 trials with purine and pyrimidine antagonists, only fluroxidine (FUDR) exhibited moderate efficacy [9, 10]. Acivicin (a glutamine antagonist from *Streptomyces sviceus*) and alanosine (an antitumor antibiotic from *Streptomyces alanosinicus*) induced PR in 4%

(95% CI = 0%–11%) and 3% (95% CI = 0%–9%) of 27 and 36 cases, respectively. Fludarabine (a purine derivative of adenosine arabinoside) was inactive (0%, 95% CI = 0%–6%) in 45 patients, as was aminothiadiazole (a purine inhibitor of inosine monophosphate dehydrogenase) with a 2% (95% CI = 0%–6%) PR rate in 46 patients. Sparfosic acid (*N*-[phosphonoacetyl]-1 aspartate or PALA), which inhibits de novo pyrimidine synthesis, produced 2 (3%, 95% CI = 0%–7%) PRs in 66 adequately treated cases, while DAC (5-aza-2-deoxycytidine) gave no (95% CI = 0%–22%) responses in 12 cases. FUDR, an old agent used primarily for intrahepatic artery infusional therapy of colorectal carcinoma, was examined in a 14-day continuous infusional chronobiological schedule of 0.15 mg/kg day. The chronobiological dosage schedule, which supposedly permits a significantly higher total daily FUDR dose than that usually tolerated, was administered in the following manner: 68% of the daily dose was administered between 1500 and 2100 h, 14% between 2100 and 0300 h, 4% between 0300 and 0900 h, and 14% between 0900 and 1500 h [10]. Initially reported were 29% CR or PR in 62 cases, but two other trials in 50 and 31 cases noted a 10% rate, and this rate increased by an additional 10% + in some studies when the primary tumor was excluded from responding sites. Nine cases had a minor response. The median durations of CR or PR were short, 5.5–7.0 months, and median survival was approximately 10 months. Whether the chronobiological schedule is important has been questioned by one study of constant continuous infusion of 0.100–0.275 mg/m^2 day for 14 days in ten, mostly pretreated, patients, of whom three (30%, 95% CI = 1%–59%) responded [9]. With an overall remission rate of 22% (95% CI = 15%–29%) in 153 patients, this agent, thus far, has demonstrated modest to moderate antitumor activity and needs to be evaluated in a randomized phase III trial.

Miscellaneous agent trials in 445 cases noted 33 (7%) CR or PR (95% CI = 5%–9%). A new trial of didemnin B, a depsipeptide marine product from sea urchins, noted one PR in 21 adequately treated cases [6], and, when combined with a prior study [10], the overall rate is 2% (95% CI = 0%–6%). Mitoguazone (a polyamine inhibitor), which had previously been tested, was further evaluated but still proved only marginally (5%) active. In a total of 180 patients, remissions occurred in 6% (95% CI = 2%–10%).

Lonidamine (a male antifertility agent because of mitochondrial hexokinase inhibition) produced PR in 8% (95% CI = 0%–19%) of 25 cases, and n-methylformamide (a polar solvent which induces differentiation) was inactive (95% CI = 0%–12%) in 27 patients. Lastly, another immunological approach combined 1, 2-benzopyrone, 100 mg po qd, with cimetidine, 300 mg q.i.d. started 15 days later. These agents were thought to modulate the immune system by increasing natural killer (NK) cell activity. Initially, there were 3 CR and 11 PR in 42 cases with remissions lasting a median of 5 months; of interest is that tumor regression occurred in only 31 nephrectomized patients compared to none in 14 who had never had resection of their primary tumor [10]. However, three other studies employing the identical schedule found 0, 0, and 3 PR in 15, 12, and 50 cases [2, 10], respectively, as well as no immunological enhancement measured by hypersensitivity skin testing, lymphocyte blastogenic response, lymphocyte number, T-cell, and T-helper and suppressor cells (Th/Ts). Therefore, the overall rate is 14% (95% CI = 8%–20%). When cimetidine was used alone or with interferon, there were 2 (8%) PR and 1 (4%) CR + 1 (4%) PR, respectively, in each of 25 unpretreated cases, the latter being a rate well within that expected for interferon used singularly.

Conclusion

Renal cell carcinoma remains a chemotherapeutically resistant tumor, and despite evaluation of over 41 new agents given in a variety of doses and schedules, either alone or in combination, in 2309 patients, the overall response rate remains marginal, 5% (95% CI = 4%–6%). Present data find CR and PR generally in the 15% range for interferon, for various interleukin-2 therapies, and for other biological response modifiers. Perhaps the combination of immunological modulators and chemotherapeutic agents may be found beneficial but there is now a real need to define more precisely the role of Mdr-1 in renal cell tumors since innovative therapies which modulate this gene are beginning to enter clinical trials. Additionally, with recent demonstration of phenotypic expression by renal cell carcinoma, evidenced by many new monoclonal antibodies, chemotherapeutic agents attached to these antibodies may yet play an important therapeutic role. Presently, it is perfectly reasonable to offer an investigational approach to patients with renal cell carcinoma since available cytotoxic chemotherapy offers no therapeutic advantage over observation alone.

References

1. Fojo AT, Shen DW, Mickley LA, et al. (1987) Intrinsic drug resistance in human kidney cancer is associated with expression of a human multidrug-resistance gene. J Clin Oncol 5: 1922–1927
2. Glynne-Jones R, Plowman N, Hendry W, Kirby R, Miller R, Harnett A (1990) Treatment of metastatic renal cell carcinoma with coumarin (1, 2-benzopyrone) and cimetidine. Proc Am Soc Clin Oncol 9 (abstract 541): 139
3. Harris DT (1983) Hormonal therapy and chemotherapy for renal cell carcinoma. Semin Oncol 10: 422–430
4. Hrushesky WJ, Murphy GP (1977) Current status of therapy for advanced renal cell carcinoma. J Surg Oncol 9: 277–288
5. Kish J, Ensley J, Al-Sarraf M (1990) Phase II evaluation of 4′deoxy-doxorubicin in advanced renal cell carcinoma. Am J Clin Oncol 13: 17–18
6. Motzer R, Scher H, Bajorin D, Sternberg C, Bosl GB (1990) Phase II trial of didemnin B in patients with advanced renal cell carcinoma. Invest New Drugs 8: 391–392
7. Stephens RL, Goodman P, Crawford ED, et al. (1990) Evaluation of menogaril in renal cell carcinoma. Invest New Drugs 8: S69–71
8. Trump DL, Elson P (1990) Evaluation of carboplatin (NSC 241240) in patients with recurrent or metastatic renal cell carcinoma. Invest New Drugs 8: 201–203
9. Wilkinson M, Stagg R, Crobman B, Carroll P, Verook A (1990) A phase II trial of constant rate FUDR infusion in patients with metastatic renal cell carcinoma. Proc Am Soc Clin Oncol 9 (Abstr 538): 139
10. Yagoda A (1989) Chemotherapy of renal cell carcinoma: 1983–1989. Semin Urol 7(4): 199–206

Modulation of Multidrug Resistance in Human Renal Cell Carcinomas

G.H. Mickisch[1] and P.M. Alken[2]

Introduction

Intrinsic chemoresistance has major impact on the dismal prognosis of patients with disseminated renal cell carcinoma (RCC) in the absence of reliable therapeutic alternatives [27]. P-170 glycoprotein was identified as a putative mechanism conferring drug resistance. Recently, a high expression of *MDR* 1 gene mRNA [13] as well as of P-170 glycoprotein [17–19] was traced in human RCCs, which may partially explain the high degree of de novo resistance. Calcium antagonists (CAs) are substances which interfere with the calcium intake at the cytoplasmatic membrane. They are mainly employed in the treatment of cardiovascular disorders such as hypertension, arrhythmia and angina pectoris. Lately, the interaction of CAs with chemotherapeutics to enhance cytotoxicity has gained particular interest. It has been shown that CAs reverse acquired resistance of experimental animal tumors [25] to some anticancer drugs and increase the life span of tumor-bearing animals compared to those merely treated with vinca alkaloids [21].

In solid human tumors like non-small-cell lung cancer [24], colon cancer [11], or glioblastomas [12], CAs potentiate the effect of vincristine. The mechanisms are not yet fully understood, but there is substantial evidence that inhibition of the energy-dependent drug efflux related to P-170 glycoprotein in multidrug resistant (MDR) cells plays an important role [2, 26].

Recent publications have demonstrated that, in at least five cases of multiple myeloma and one case of non-Hodgkin's lymphoma,

[1] Laboratory of Molecular Biology, National Cancer Institute, National Institutes of Health, Bethesda, MD 20892, USA
[2] Urologische Klinik, Klinikum Mannheim der Universität Heidelberg, Theodor-Kutzer-Ufer, W-6800 Mannheim, FRG

G. Staehler S. Pomer (Eds.)
Basic and Clinical Research on Renal Cell Carcinoma

clinical drug resistance is associated with P-170 glycoprotein expression, and that the addition of verapamil (VPM) can partially reverse chemoresistance [5]. Vinblastine (VBL) is accepted as the most potent single cytostatic in RCCs [27] even though its clinical use is very limited at present as not more than 20% of the patients with metastatic RCC show a response. We were, therefore, interested in evaluating the effects of VBL in combination with certain CAs in primary human RCCs. We selected representatives of four major classes of calcium-blocking agents [23] such as VPM (racemic form), nifedipine (NIF), diltiazem (DIL) and flunarizine (FLU). In addition, we assessed R-verapamil (R-VPM), the R(+)-stereoisomer of VPM, since it revealed a tenfold lower cardiovascular activity than racemic VPM [6], as well as nitrendipine (NIT) and nimodipine (NIM), modern derivatives of NIF.

Materials and Methods

Fresh tumor specimens from 32 primary human RCCs were placed in chilled Hank's balanced salt solution (HBSS, Seromed, Berlin, FRG) and processed under sterile conditions within 1 h after nephrectomy. Aliquots of the tumor probes served to determine the degree of chemoresistance and for examining the reversal of drug resistance by calcium antagonists, or were shock-frozen in liquid nitrogen and preserved below −80°C for further immunohistochemical studies.

Microculture Tetrazolium Test

The basic feature of the microculture tetrazolium test (MTT) test is the cell-generated conversion of a yellow tetrazolium salt into a purple-colored formazan precipitate. This reaction directly indicates cell viability [1]. Single cell suspensions were prepared by mechanical disaggregation, tumor cells were filtrated through textile multilayer gauze, and purified by Ficoll density centrifugation. Then, the MTT was carried out as previously described [16, 18, 19].

Statistical analysis included the Student's *t*-test, and the Bonferroni–Holm correction for curves was applied [10].

Demonstration of P-170 Glycoprotein

Cryostat cuts (6 µm) of the RCCs were air-dried and fixed in acetone. The primary monoclonal antibody (moab) C 219 (Centocor, Brussels,

Belgium) [15] was applied (5–20 µg/ml 2 h). After washing, the tumor tissues were incubated with biotinylated sheep anti-(mouse) immunoglobulin second antibody (dilution 1:50, 30 min; Amersham, Braunschweig, FRG) and the streptavidine biotinylated horseradish peroxidase complex binding (Amersham) (dilution 1:100, 30 min) was carried out. Peroxidase activity was visualized by 3-amino-9-ethylcarbazole/H_2O_2 (5–10 min). Counterstaining was performed with hematoxilyn. Negative trials were run without a primary antibody. MDR/CHO (Chinese Hamster Ovary) cells served as positive control groups. The tissues were scored as positive or negative in accordance with the color reaction. A minimum of ten different cryostat sections from various parts of the tumor were analyzed. Although the staining reaction appeared focal rather than diffuse, and the color intensity varied, a positive signal at the cytoplasmic membrane was, when present, clearly visible in positive samples. The decision, however, to regard a tumor as definitely negative was based on the absence of positive staining in any cell of any part of the tumor examined.

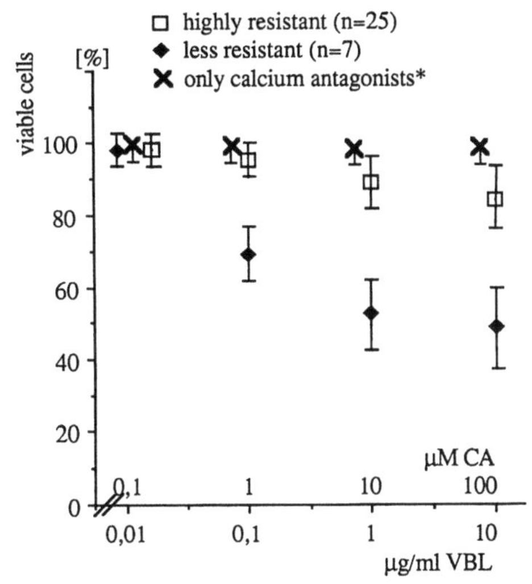

Fig. 1. Determination of the degree of chemoresistance in human renal cell carcinomas (RCCs) (n = 32) using a microculture tetrazolium test (MTT). Values expressed as a percentage of viable tumor cells as compared to untreated groups. Vinblastine (*VBL*) was applied in final concentrations from 0.01–10 µg/ml cell suspension for 16 h incubation time. MTT was then added for a further 4 h and optical density measured at 540 nm. The effect of calcium antagonists (CAs) was studied in final concentrations ranging from 0.1–100 μM under the same conditions

All reagents were of p.a. grade and were, if not otherwise stated, purchased from Boehringer Mannheim, FRG.

Results

Twenty five of 32 RCCs proved to be highly refractory to VBL in the MTT microculture assay (Fig. 1), e.g., the number of viable tumor cells in the presence of this chemotherapeutic agent did not distinctly differ from that of the untreated control group, whereas in seven cases (Fig. 1), a clear reduction was measured. This division into highly and less resistant tumors is significant for concentrations equal to or greater than 0.1 μg/ml VBL ($p < 0.001$). All CAs examined in concentrations of up to 100 μ*M* did not affect the ability of RCCs to produce MTT formazans (Fig. 1).

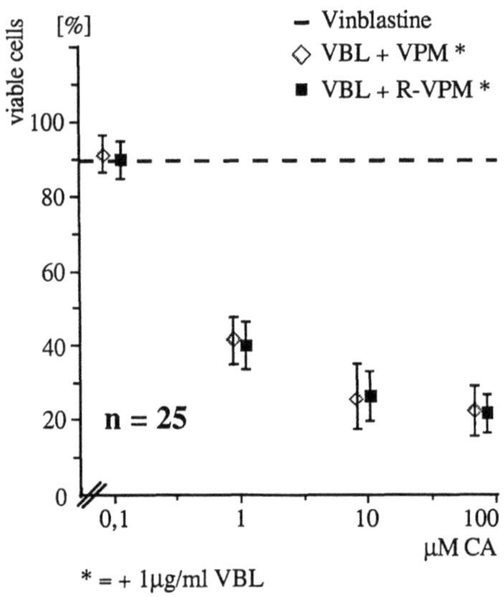

Fig. 2. Reversal of chemoresistance by verapamil (*VPM*) and R-verapamil (*R-VPM*) in human renal cell carcinomas (RCCs) (n = 25, group of highly-resistant tumors from Fig. 1). Values expressed as a percentage of viable tumor cells exposed to different concentrations of calcium antagonists (*CA*s) and to a constant concentration of 1 μg/ml vinblastine (*VBL*) as compared to groups which only contain the same amount of chemotherapeutic agent. The *dotted line* indicates the effect of 1 μg/ml VBL alone on this group of RCCs, data derived from Fig. 1

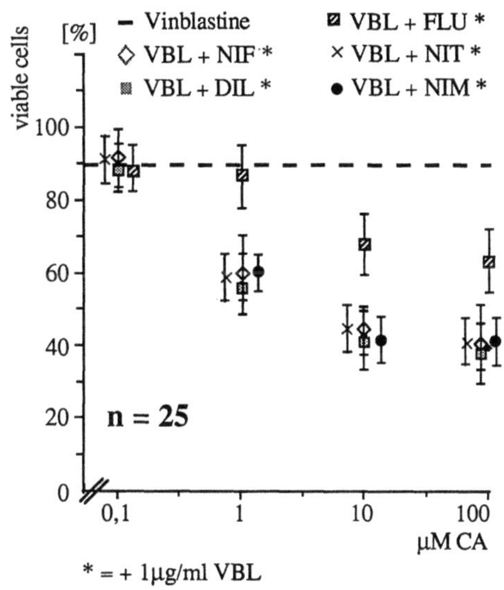

Fig. 3. Reversal of chemoresistance by calcium antagonists (*CA*s) in human renal cell carcinomas (RCCs) ($n = 25$, group of highly-resistant tumors from Fig. 1). Values expressed as a percentage of viable tumor cells exposed to different concentrations of calcium antagonists and to a constant concentration of 1 μg/ml vinblastine (*VBL*) as compared to groups which only contain the same amount of chemotherapeutic agent. The *dotted line* indicates the effect of 1 μg/ml VBL alone on this group of renal cell carcinomas (RCCs), data derived from Fig. 1

The combined application of calcium antagonists and VBL, however, led to a varying significant decrease of viable tumor cells (Figs. 2, 3), depending on the substance applied. The strongest reversal of chemoresistance was obtained with VPM or R-VPM ($p < 0.001$) (Fig. 2), whereas FLU displayed only minor effects (Fig. 3).

NIF, NIT, NIM and DIL exhibited similar behavior and reached about 70% of the VPM/R-VPM activity. High conformity between NIF and its derivatives, NIT and NIM, as well as between VPM and R-VPM, was ascertained (Figs. 2, 3). Furthermore, Fig. 2 and Fig. 3 demonstrate that a minimum concentration of 1 μ*M* VPM/R-VPM, NIF or DIL was required to halve tumor cell viability in the presence of 1 μg/ml VBL. The data indicate that all primary RCCs were influenced by VBL + VPM/R-VPM, but also by DIL and NIF.

The degree of VBL potentiation by CAs showed a positive correlation to the extent of intrinsic chemoresistance to this drug, i.e., the highest enhancement was obtained in the RCCs most refractory

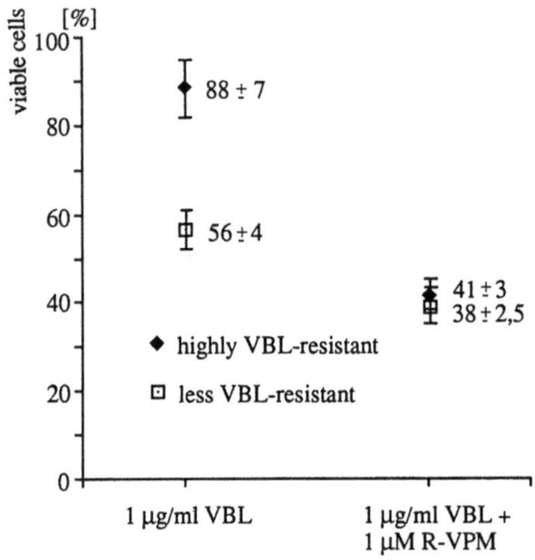

Fig. 4. Effect of 1 µg/ml vinblastine (*VBL*) in combination with 1 µ*M* R-verapamil (*R-VPM*) on human renal cell carcinomas (RCCs) with regard to the degree of chemoresistance "highly resistant" (n = 25), "less-resistant" (n = 7) as detailed in Fig. 1. Values expressed as a percentage of viable tumor cells exposed to untreated control groups to determine the effect of VBL and of control groups containing 1 µg/ml VBL of measure the effect of R-VPM

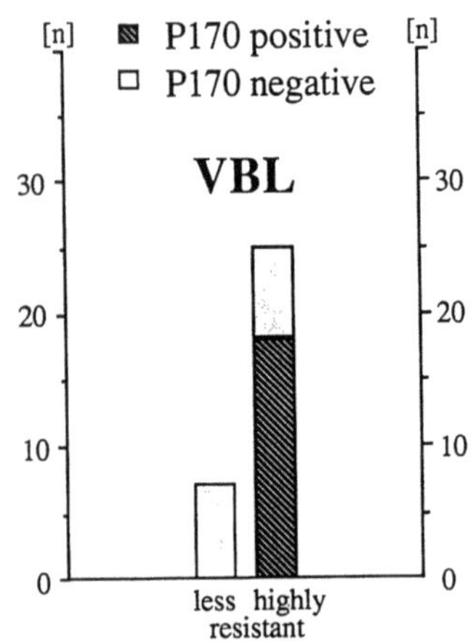

Fig. 5. Detection of P-170 glycoprotein in human renal cell carcinomas (RCCs) (n = 32) using Moab C219 in relation to the chemoresistance pattern. Chemoresistance data derived from Fig. 1

to drug treatment and vice versa. The accumulated results regarding R-VPM have been depicted in Fig. 4.

P-170 glycoprotein was traced in 18 out of 32 RCCs using moab C 219. Of the highly resistant tumors, 72% expressed this specific resistance characteristic, but none of the less resistant cases did so (Fig. 5). Eight of 10 well-differentiated (G1) [9] and 10 of 16 quite well differentiated (G2) RCCs were detected to be P-170 positive, but none of 6 undifferentiated (G3) tumors (data not shown) were.

Discussion

So far, clinical trials for enhancing the cytotoxicity of various chemotherapeutic agents by the combination with VPM have not been very rewarding. The limiting factor proved to be the inherent cardiovascular activity of racemic VPM with subsequent hypotension and/or prolonged atrioventricular conduction time. No objective tumor remissions after i.v. injection [22], or only partial responses after oral administration of VPM [4, 20], were observed. One possible explanation for the differing clinical results in consequence of the route of administration may be that higher doses can be tolerated after oral uptake of racemic VPM [8]. This fact has been attributed to the inherent properties of the components of racemic VPM. On i.v. administration, both stereoisomers (R-VPM + L-VPM) exert their effects simultaneously, whereas on oral administration, R-VPM as well as the metabolite norverapamil become efficacious first owing to diverse resorption and to a different so-called "first-pass" effect in the liver [7]. However, R-VPM reveals ten fold lower cardiovascular activity than racemic VPM [6].

The experimental data on human RCCs show that in vitro concentrations of at least 1 μM VPM are required to enhance the effect of VBL significantly (Fig. 2). These concentrations are difficult to realize in vivo [8]. Therefore, the clinical application of chemosensitizing agents such as CAs requires reduced cardiovascular activity of the CAs while they maintain their influence on chemoresistance. Among the evaluated CAs, only the newly available isomer R-VPM (Figs. 2, 3) fulfills these criteria with adequate potentiation of VBL cytotoxicity (Fig. 2) and with ten fold lower cardiovascular activity [6]. But even in high concentrations of up to 100 μM, none of the CAs evaluated overcame VBL resistance totally in any of the 32 human RCCs, and a substantial percentage of tumor cells survived (Figs. 2, 3).

Apparently, undifferentiated RCCs in this series appear to respond with a stronger decrease of viable tumor cells under the influence of VBL than G1 or G2 tumors. The explanation for this could be the lack of P-170 expression in these cases (Fig. 5). In fact, P-170 expression seems to prevail in G1 and G2 tumors. Indirect support may be deduced from previous reports referring to 42 RCCs displaying a correlation between tumor grading and the expression of *MDR* 1 RNA. Elevated levels were traced in well-differentiated RCCs in contrast to poorly differentiated carcinomas [14]. Furthermore, the reversal of chemoresistance effected by quinidine in human RCCs showed a relationship to elevated *MDR* 1 RNA levels [14]. Our data using different CAs suggest that the circumvention of resistance was more pronounced in those cases which exhibited the resistance characteristic P-170. However, the fact that the enhancement of VBL cytotoxicity by CAs could even be detected in tumors where P-170 could not be traced may lead to the interpretation that the applied immunohistochemical method may be limited to P-170 overexpression, and low P-170 levels may be missed as demonstrated in human cell lines [3].

References

1. Alley MC, Scudiero DA, Monks A, et al. (1988) Feasibility of drug screening with panels of human tumor cell lines using a microculture tetrazolium assay. Cancer Res 48: 589–601
2. Baeyens JM (1988) Interactions between calcium channel blockers and non-cardiovascular drugs: Interactions with anticancer drugs. Pharmacol Toxicol 63: 1–7
3. Broxterman HJ, Pinedo HM, Kuiper CM, et al. (1989) Immunohistochemical detection of P-glycoprotein in human tumor cells with a low degree of drug resistance. Int J Cancer 43: 340–341
4. Cantwell B, Puamah P, Harris AL (1985) Phase I and phase II study of oral verapamil (VRP) and intravenous vindesine (VDN). Br J Cancer 52: 425
5. Dalton WS, Grogan TM, Meltzer PS, et al. (1989) Drug-resistance in multiple myeloma and non-Hodgkin's Lymphoma: Detection of P-glycoprotein and potential circumvention by addition of verapamil to chemotherapy. J Clin Oncol 7: 415–424
6. Echizen H, Brecht T, Niedergesaess S, Vogelgesang B, Eichelbaum M (1985) The effect of dextro-laevo- and racemic verapamil on atrio-ventricular conduction in humans. Am Heart J 109: 210–217
7. Eichelbaum M, Birkel P, Grube E, Gutgemann U, Somerogyi A (1980) Effects on P-R intervals in relation to verapamil plasma levels following single i.v. and oral administration and during chronic treatment. Klin Wochenschr 58: 919–925

8. Hamann SR, Blouin RA, McAllister Jr RG (1984) Clinical pharmacokinetics of verapamil. Clinical Pharmacokinetics 9: 26–41
9. Hermanek P (1987) UICC, TNM Classification of malignant tumors, 4th edn. Springer, Berlin Heidelberg New York Tokyo
10. Holm S (1979) A simple sequentially rejective multiple test procedure. Scand J Statist 6: 65–70
11. Ince P, Appleton DR, Finney KJ, Sunter JP, Watson AJ (1986) Verapamil increases the sensitivity of primary human colorectal carcinoma tissue to vincristine. Br J Cancer 53: 137–139
12. Kaba K, Tanki E, Morimura T, Matsumoto T (1985) Potentiation of vincristine effects in human and murine gliomas by calcium channel blockers or calmodulin inhibitors. J Neurosurg 63: 905–911
13. Kakehi Y, Kanamaru H, Yoshida O, Ohkubo H, Nakanishi S, Gottesman MM, Pastan I (1988) Measurements of multidrug resistance messenger-RNA in urogenital cancers; elevated expression in renal cell carcinoma is associated with intrinsic drug resistance. J Urol 139: 862–865
14. Kanamaru H, Kakehi Y, Yoshia O, Nakanishi S, Pastan I, Gottesman MM (1989) MDR1 RNA levels in human renal cell carcinomas: correlation with grade and prediction of reversal of doxorubicin resistance by quinidine in tumor explants. J Natl Cancer Inst 81: 844–849
15. Kartner N, Evernden-Porelle D, Bradley G, Ling V (1985) Detection of P-170 glycoprotein in multidrug-resistant cell lines by monoclonal antibodies. Nature 316: 820–823
16. Mickisch G, Fajta S, Keilhauer G, Schlick E, Tschada R, Alken P (1990) Chemosensitivity testing of primary human renal cell carcinoma by a tetrazolium based microculture assay (MTT). Urol Res 18: 131–136
17. Mickisch G, Bier H, Bergler W, Bak M, Tschada R, Alken P (1990) P-170 glycoprotein, glutathione and associated enzymes in relation to chemoresistance of primary human renal cell carcinomas. Urol Intern 45: 170–176
18. Mickisch G, Kössig J, Keilhauer G, Schlick E, Tschada R, Alken P (1990) Effects of calcium antagonists in multidrug resistant primary human renal call carcinomas. Cancer Res 50: 3670–3674
19. Mickisch G, Röhrich K, Kössig J, Forster S, Tschada R, Alken P (1990) Mechanisms and modulation of multidrug resistance in primary human renal cell carcinoma. J Urol 144: 755–759
20. Milroy R, Connory L, Banham F, Hutcheon D, Maclntyre D, Stack B (1987) Randomized trial of verapamil in addition to chemotherapy for small cell lung cancer. Thorax 42: 209
21. Morrow M, Wait RB, Rosenthal RA, Gamelli RL (1987) Verpamil enhances antitumor activity without increasing myeloid toxicity. Surgery 101: 63–65
22. Ozols RF, Cunnian RE, Klecker RW, Hamilton FC, Ostchega Y, Parillo JE, Young RC (1987) Verapamil and adriamycine in the treatment of drug-resistant ovarian cancer patients. J Clin Oncol 5: 641–647
23. Paoletti R, Govoni S (1987) Classification of calcium antagonists: Proposal of the WHO Committee. Pharmacol Res Comm Vol. 19, 3: 195–209
24. Simmonds AP, Moyes P, Nicol A, Davidson KG, Faichney A (1986) Enhancement of cytotoxicity of vindesine and cis-platinum for human lung tumours by the use of verapamil in vitro. Br J Cancer 54: 1015–1018

25. Tsuruo T (1983) Reversal of acquired resistance to vinca alcaloids and anthracycline antibiotics. Cancer Treat Rep 67: 889–894
26. Tsuruo T (1988) Mechanisms of multidrug resistance and implications for therapy. Jpn J Cancer Res (Gann) 79: 285–296
27. Vugrin D (1987) Systematic therapy of metastatic renal cell carcinoma. Sem Nephrol 7: 152–162

Transgenic Mice Carrying the Human MDR 1 Gene: Reliable In Vivo Probes to Examine Multidrug Resistance

G.H. Mickisch[1], M.M. Gottesman[2], and I. Pastan[1]

Introduction

Resistance to chemotherapy poses an ultimate obstacle to curing human cancer which is not amenable to definitive surgical or radiation treatment. Numerous investigations have uncovered processes instigating a clinically relevant broad cross-resistance spectrum to natural product cytotoxic compounds without striking functional or structural similarities, termed multiple drug resistance (MDR) [15]. The compiled evidence implies that the so-called multidrug transporter, P-170 glycoprotein, encoded by the human *MDR* 1 gene [23], is sufficient to produce MDR of cancer cells [8]. Its functions predominantly involve the rapid extrusion of hydrophobic chemotherapeutic agents from the cell before they can exert their designated actions [11].

Recently, it became evident that most drug-resistant human tumors express the characteristics of MDR [7], and the presence or absence of this factor clearly predicts the clinical outcome of chemotherapeutic regimens [2].

Subsequently, MDR has evolved from a laboratory novelty to a phenomenon with potentially high clinical importance. One aspect of MDR has attracted particular attention: A multitude of chemosensitizers reverse MDR by inhibiting the P-170 related efflux pump [3].

Initial reports on a limited number of patients claim to have traced similar activity in clinical trials [4]. However, inherent side effects impeding sufficient dosage in vivo still necessitate the continuous search for new resistance modifiers [9].

[1] Laboratories of Molecular Biology and [2] Cell Biology, National Cancer Institute, National Institutes of Health, Bethesda, MD 20892, USA

G. Staehler S. Pomer (Eds.)
Basic and Clinical Research on Renal Cell Carcinoma

In order to further substantiate in vitro studies of MDR in a suitable preclinical in vivo model, our laboratory has engineered transgenic mice carrying the human *MDR* 1 gene under the control of a chicken β-actin promoter [6]. The preliminary characterization exhibited *MDR* 1 expression primarily in bone marrow in amounts corresponding to those found in human tumors. Furthermore, we traced the translation of *MDR* 1 gene to the protein level indicated by detection of P-170 glycoprotein, and gained a first hint regarding the functional capacity of the inserted gene, since daunomycin (DAU) chemotherapy did not alter the peripheral white blood count (WBC).

The studies reported here investigate the functional protection of a circumscribed organ like bone marrow by the human *MDR* 1 gene against a variety of chemotherapeutic drugs presently in clinical use and focus on the reversal of MDR effected by chemosensitizers applicable in humans.

Materials and Methods

MDR-Transgenic Mice

The construction of the original plasmid carrying the full-length cDNA coding region of *MDR* 1 [16] and the injection of this cDNA under control of a chicken β-actin promoter using standard techniques [10] have been described elsewhere [6].

Homozygous males from the line MDR-39 [6] were backcrossed to MDR-negative females of the progenitor line C57BL/6 × SJL F1. The resulting MDR-heterozygous descendants were carefully analyzed for the expression of the human *MDR* 1 gene using tail samples [10] in accordance with Southern's method [19] and hybridized with a MDR-specific probe generated in this laboratory [20]. In these studies, 6- to 8-week-old, sex-matched litter mates were investigated exclusively.

Test Conditions

Cisplatin (CP) and etoposide (ETO) were obtained from Bristol-Myers Comp., Syracuse. All other chemotherapeutic agents as well as quinine (Q) and quinidine (QD) were purchased from Sigma Chemical Comp., St. Louis; verapamil (VPM) and R(+)-stereoisomer of verapamil (R-VPM) were provided by courtesy of BASF Bio-research Corp., Cambridge. The drugs were administered intraperitoneally in the lower right quadrant of the abdominal cavity. In studies involving the combined application of chemosensitizers and cytotoxic agents, the putative resistance modifiers were injected 20 min prior to chemotherapy. Drug concentrations were adjusted to respect a maximum volume of 400 µl per therapy applying a single dose treatment schedule. Experiments included a minimum of three animals per group, and were repeated at least once.

Measurements

Peripheral blood was collected by periorbital bleeding with heparinized microhematocrit capillary tubes (Fisher Scientific Corp., Pittsburgh) and diluted 1:20 (vol/vol) in 3% acetic acid solution for erythrocyte lysis. The refractile, viable leukocytes (WBC) were counted on an ultra-plane Neubauer's hemocytometer (Hausser Scientific, Pittsburgh, PA). Hematocrit was measured by centrifuging (12 000 × *g*; 5 min) another heparinized microcapillary tube and expressing the value as a ratio of the length of the red cell column to that of the whole blood column. Differential WBC and approximate number of thrombocytes were obtained by exposing (staining rack) air-dried whole blood smears to modified Wright stain (Accustain, Sigma; 5 min) by neutralizing in phosphate buffer (pH 7.2, 5 min), and by washing in distilled water (10 min). Subsequently, the blood film was analyzed using an oil immersion lens.

Results

The injection of all chemotherapeutic agents examined causes a dramatic reduction of the WBC of more than 50% in normal mice as compared to untreated controls (Fig. 1). In MDR-transgenic mice, however, the bone marrow is apparently protected against the same concentrations of either vinca alkaloids, anthracyclines, antibiotics or epipodophyllotoxins, but not against CP, methotrexate (MTX) or 5-fluorouracil (5FU; Fig. 1).

Analyzing the results of chemotherapy on the differential WBC, it becomes evident that neutrophil granulocytes were more frequently affected than lymphocytes (Table 1). Thrombocyte numbers were only moderately influenced, and none of the animals exhibited bleeding during the experiments. No alteration of the hematocrit was noted (Table 1).

Table 1. Hematological parameters in MDR-transgenic mice or negative siblings in accordance with daunomycin chemotherapy (10 mg/kg). Experiments were conducted on 6 female, 7-week old litter mates, as explained in Materials and Methods

	Day 0		Day 5		Day 5 MDR+	
	Normal	MDR+	Normal	MDR+	VPM (30 mg/kg)	R-VPM (150 mg/kg)
WBC	8.9	9.1	2.7	9.6	2.6	1.2
($\times 10^3/\mu l$)	(7.0–10.5)	(7.3–10.7)	(2.5–2.8)	(8.3–11.2)	(2.5–2.7)	(0.5–1.7)
Neutrophils	4.9	3.1	1.2	4.6	0.9	4.9
(band forms) (%)	(2–6)	(1–5)	(0–3)	(2–8)	(0–3)	(2–7)
Neutrophils	21.4	23.9	5.1	24.7	4.7	16.8
(%)	(18–24)	(19–30)	(1–8)	(21–30)	(1–7)	(13–21)
Lymphocytes	67.7	67.2	74.7	64	78.2	60.1
(%)	(61–70)	(61–70)	(68–78)	(60–69)	(70–82)	(54–65)
Basophils	1.5	1.3	2.4	1.5	1.6	1.0
(%)	(0–3)	(0–3)	(0–3)	(0–3)	(1–3)	(0–3)
Eosinophils	0.2	0.4	0.8	0.4	0.6	0.2
(%)	(0–2)	(0–2)	(0–3)	(0–2)	(0–2)	(0–2)
Monocytes	4.0	3.1	6.2	2.7	4.1	2.8
(%)	(1–8)	(1–6)	(2–9)	(1–6)	(2–8)	(1–5)
others	0.3	1	9.6	2.1	9.9	14.2
(%)	(0–3)	(0–3)	(5–12)	(1–4)	(6–13)	(9–17)
Thrombocytes	245	230	175	225	180	155
($\times 10^3/\mu l$)	(160–400)	(155–410)	(120–280)	(150–420)	(110–260)	(100–190)
Hematocrit	48	47	50	46	49	49
(%)	(44–51)	(44–51)	(47–52)	(44–50)	(46–52)	(46–51)

Values are means; range is indicated in parentheses.

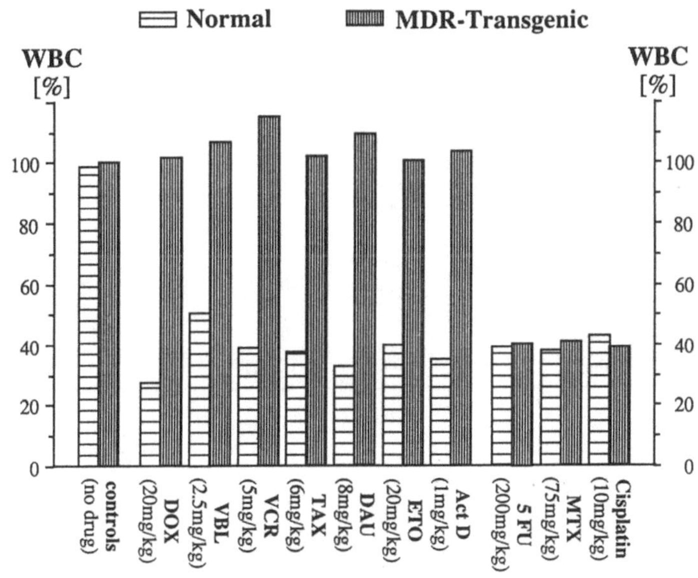

Fig. 1. Bone marrow toxicity of chemotherapeutic agents for normal and MDR-transgenic mice. Drugs were administered i.p. in a single dose on day 0. Values are expressed as a ratio of WBC on day 5 to day 0. Experiments included a minimum of three animals per group and were repeated at least once. Dosage was selected to insure a significant (>50%) reduction of WBC in normal mice without causing generalized toxicity

Higher doses of cytotoxic drugs lead to a stronger decrease of the WBC in normal mice. The data for taxol (TAX) are depicted in Fig. 2a. Obviously, the lowest number of leukocytes was detected on day 5, whereas on day 7 a minor rise could already be ascertained. Chemosensitizers like VPM, Q or QD, even in high concentrations, illicit no effect on the WBC (Fig. 2a). By itself, 10 mg/kg of TAX does not change the WBC in MDR-transgenic mice (Fig. 2a–d), whereas in contrast to the former the combined application of TAX and Q (Fig. 2b), TAX and QD (Fig. 2c) or TAX and VPM (Fig. 2d) exerts considerable bone marrow toxicity.

Standard resistance modifiers like VPM, Q or QD function in a dose-dependent fashion in MDR-transgenic mice. High concentrations lower the WBC to levels equivalent to those reached by DAU-chemotherapy alone in unprotected normal animals (Fig. 3a–c).

Applying 150 mg/kg of the newly available R-VPM demonstrates that even in MDR-negative normal mice DAU-associated bone marrow toxicity can be further potentiated (Fig. 4b). R-VPM alone does not

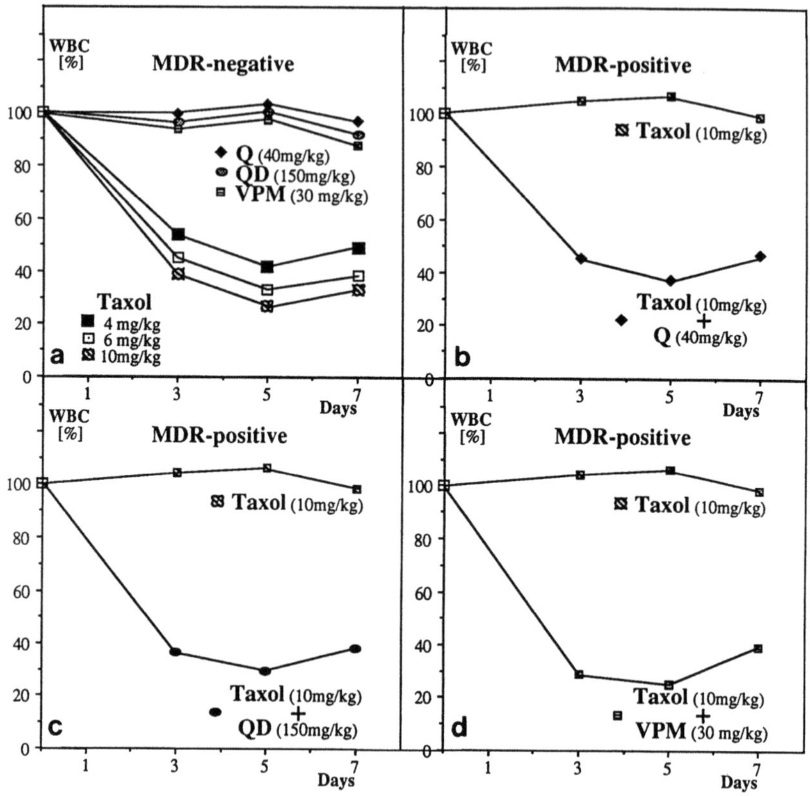

Fig. 2a–d. Time dependent effects of taxol and/or chemosensitizers on the WBC of mice. **a** Normal mice. **b** MDR-transgenic mice; TAX alone or combined with Q. **c** MDR-transgenic mice; TAX alone or combined with QD. **d** MDR-transgenic mice; TAX alone or combined with VPM. Experiments were conducted as explained in Materials and Methods and in the legend to Fig. 1

Fig. 3a–c. Dose-dependent reversal of bone marrow protection against daunomycin effected by the human *MDR* 1 gene. **a** DAU (10 mg/kg) combined with VPM. **b** DAU (10 mg/kg) combined with QD. **c** DAU (10 mg/kg) combined with Q. Experiments were conducted as explained in Materials and Methods and in the legend to Fig. 1

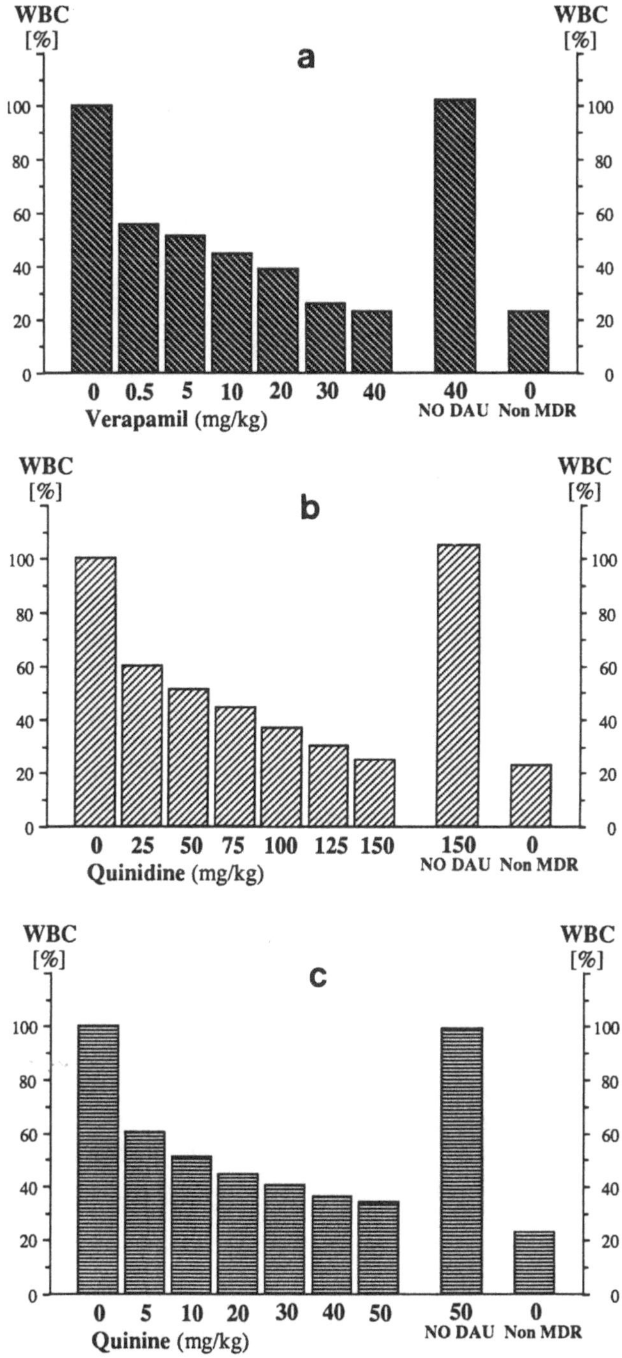
WBC
[%]
a
0
20
40
60
80
100
0 0.5 5 10 20 30 40
Verapamil (mg/kg)
40
NO DAU
0
Non MDR
b
0 25 50 75 100 125 150
Quinidine (mg/kg)
150
NO DAU
0
Non MDR
c
0 5 10 20 30 40 50
Quinine (mg/kg)
50
NO DAU
0
Non MDR

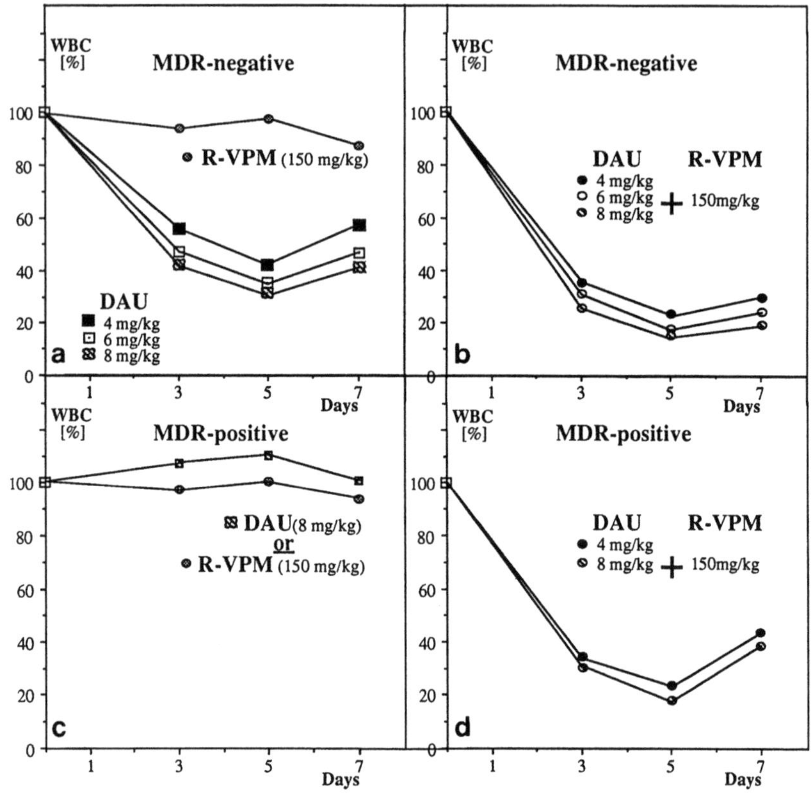

Fig. 4a–d. Toxicity of daunomycin alone or in combination with R(+)-verapamil to the bone marrow of mice. **a** Normal mice; DAU *or* R-VPM (150 mg/kg). **b** Normal mice; DAU *and* R-VPM (150 mg/kg). **c** MDR-transgenic mice; DAU *or* R-VPM (150 mg/kg). **d** MDR-transgenic mice; DAU *and* R-VPM (150 mg/kg). Experiments were conducted as explained in Materials and Methods and in the legend to Fig. 1

diminish the leucocyte count (Fig. 4a). In MDR-transgenic animals, R-VPM circumvents bone marrow resistance (Fig. 4c) against 8 mg/kg or 4 mg/kg doses of DAU (Fig. 4d), respectively.

Moreover, 0.5 mg/kg of VPM or 20 mg/kg of Q measurably subdue DAU resistance (Fig. 5a), whereas the combination of VPM and Q reveals additive effects (Fig. 5b).

Discussion

Several MDR-transgenic founder mice inheriting the transgene in a dominant mendelian fashion have been developed in our laboratory.

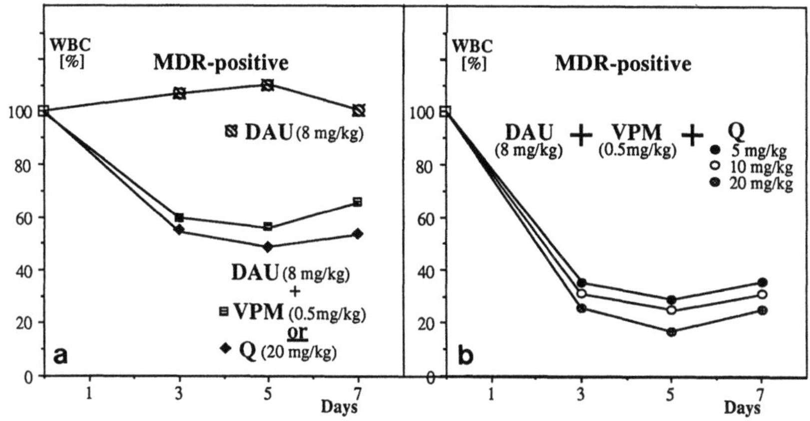

Fig. 5a, b. Additive effects of verapamil plus quinine combined with daunomycin in MDR-transgenic mice. **a** DAU alone or combined with VPM (0.5 mg/kg) *or* Q (20 mg/kg) **b** DAU (8 mg/kg) combined with VPM (0.5 mg/kg) *and* Q. Experiments were conducted as explained in Materials and Methods and in the legend to Fig. 1

We became particularly interested in line MDR-39, characterized in these studies, since our early data [6] suggested a low copy number of the *MDR* 1 construct and expression predominantly in bone marrow. Bone marrow suppression is a limiting drawback of chemotherapy.

On addressing the functional efficacy of the inserted human *MDR* 1 gene and in order to refute or confirm the in vitro specificity of the multidrug transporter [8], a panel of chemotherapeutic agents was tested in vivo (Fig. 1). When selecting drug concentrations which guarantee a significant (>50%) decrease of the periperal WBC in normal mice without exhibiting any generalized toxicity, it was shown that the human *MDR* 1 gene protects the mouse bone marrow completely against cytotoxic compounds involved in the MDR phenotype. However, substances such as CP, MTX or 5FU, which are not handled by the MDR efflux pump, caused severe bone marrow depression in both normal and transgenic animals.

Looking at the differential WBCs, the compiled evidence (Table 1) suggests that the created MDR bone marrow protection does not permit DAU to preferably affect neutrophils as in normal mice, and that the prototype chemosensitizer VPM can apparently restore a situation present in the negative progenitor line.

In consequence, we focused on the in vivo reversal of MDR. The model examined uniquely features the isolated MDR protection of a circumscribed organ, bone marrow. Therefore, we concentrated on chemotherapeutic agents already clinically known to exert mainly bone marrow toxicity like DAU [12] or TAX [18]. Among the common properties shared by compounds overcoming drug resistance in vitro [22] is the lack of stereospecificity. However, differences in inherent side effects in vivo as regards the clinical applicability require further studies, since it was considered feasible to exploit this fact in clinical trials [14]. The R(+)-stereoisomer of VPM exhibited similar potency to circumvent MDR in vitro as the standard resistance modifier, racemic (+/−) VPM, but allows much higher doses to be applied in vivo owing to reduced cardiovascular activities [5]. In addition, we investigated other basic chemosensitizers, the true stereoisomers QD and Q.

In fact, it was easy to detect that these substances potentiated bone marrow toxicity of TAX (Fig. 2b–d) and DAU (Fig. 4d) in a dose-dependent manner (Fig. 3a–c), thus rendering individual comparisons possible. Interestingly, the amount of chemotherapeutic agent applied (Fig. 4d) does not limit the chemosensitizing effect of R-VPM as long as the dose of DAU administered is sufficient to influence the WBC in unprotected mice (Fig. 4a).

Using extremely high concentrations of R-VPM (Fig. 4b, d), the combined treatment exceeds the bone marrow suppression produced by DAU alone. Analyzing differential WBCs (Table 1) may offer an explanation. Obviously, the sensitization of otherwise more resistant lymphocytes to chemotherapy has impact on the further decrease of the leucocyte number (Fig. 4b). Recently, some bone marrow cells, predominantly lymphocyte precursors, were found to express intrinsic MDR [13].

To gain additional information on the sensitivity of the MDR transgenic model system, clinically relevant concentrations of VPM and Q were assessed and shown to measurably interfere with MDR bone marrow protection against DAU (Fig. 5a). Combined application of equal doses of these chemosensitizers resulted in additive reversal of MDR (Fig. 5b). Taking the current knowledge as to how these substances may function [1] into consideration, it may be assumed that Q and VPM do not compete for the same binding site on P-170 glycoprotein. The exact mechanism is presently under investigation in our laboratory. Clinically, however, VPM plus Q is of potential interest, since intrinsic cardiovascular properties of standard resistance modifiers proved to be a major pitfall in experimental therapeutic trials to inactivate MDR so far [9]. Therefore, the association with cardiac dysfunction appears to preclude the clinical combination of antiarrhythmic drugs like QD or amiodarone, but not of the antimalarial Q [21] with the prototype chemosensitizer VPM.

References

1. Akiyama S, Cornwell MM, Kuwano M, Pastan I, Gottesman MM (1988) Most drugs that reverse multidrug resistance also inhibit photoaffinity labeling of P-glycoprotein by a vinblastine analog. Mol Pharmacol 33: 144–147
2. Chan HSL, Thorner PS, Haddad G, Ling V (1990) Immunohistochemical detection of P-glycoprotein: Prognostic correlation in soft tissue sarcoma of childhood. J Clin Oncol 8: 689–704
3. Cornwell MM, Pastan I, Gottesman MM (1987) Certain calcium channel blockers bind specifically to multidrug-resistant human KB carcinoma membrane vesicles and inhibit drug binding to P-glycoprotein. J Biol Chem 262: 2166–2170
4. Dalton WS, Grogan TM, Meltzer PS, et al. (1989) Drug resistance in multiple myeloma and non-Hodgkin's lymphoma: Detection of P-glycoprotein and potential circumvention by addition of verapamil to chemotherapy. J Clin Oncol 7: 415–424
5. Echizen H, Brecht T, Niedergesaess S, Vogelgesang B, Eichelbaum M (1985) The effect of dextro-levo- and racemic verapamil on atrioventricular conduction in humans. Am Heart J 109: 210–217
6. Galski H, Sullivan M, Willingham MC, Khew-Voon C, Gottesman MM, Pastan I, Merlino GT (1989) Expression of a human multidrug resistance cDNA (MDR-1) in the bone marrow of transgenic mice: Resistance to daunomycin induced leukopenia. Mol Cell Biol 9: 4357–4363
7. Goldstein LJ, Galski H, Fojo A, et al. (1989) Expression of the multidrug resistance gene in human cancers. J Natl Cancer Inst 81: 116–124
8. Gottesman MM and Pastan I (1988) The multidrug transporter, a double-edged sword. J Biol Chem 263: 12163–12166
9. Gottesman MM, Pastan I (1989) Clinical trials of agents that reverse multidrug resistance Editorial, J Clin Oncol 7: 409–411
10. Hogan B, Constantini F, Lacy E (1986) Manipulating the mouse embryo: a laboratory manual. Cold Spring Harbor Laboratory, Cold Spring Harbor, NY
11. Horio M, Gottesman MM, Pastan I (1988) ATP-dependent transport of vinblastine in vesicles from human multidrug resistant cells. Proc Natl Acad Sci USA 85: 3580–3584
12. Maral RJ, Jouanne M (1981) Toxicology of daunorubicin in animals and man. Cancer Treat Rep 65(Suppl 4): 9–18
13. Marie J-P, Brophy NA, Ehsan MN, Chao NJ, Sicic BI (1990) Expression of the multidrug resistance gene (mdr 1) detected by RNA phenotyping and in situ RNA hybridization in bone marrow cells. Proc AACR 31: 2198
14. Mickisch GH, Kössig J, Keilhauer G, Schlick E, Tschada RK, Alken PM (1990) Effects of calcium antagonists in multidrug resistant primary human renal cell carcinomas. Cancer Res 50: 3670–3674
15. Pastan I, Gottesman MM (1987) Multiple drug resistance in human cancer. N Engl J Med 316: 1388–1393

16. Pastan I, Gottesman MM, Ueda K, Lovelace E, Rutherford AV, Willingham MC (1988) A retrovirus carrying an MDR1 cDNA confers multidrug resistance and polarized expression of P-glycoprotein in MDCK cells. Proc Natl Acad Sci USA 85: 4486–4490
17. Robinson IB, Chin JE, Choi K, et al. (1986) Isolation of human mdr sequences amplified in multidrug-resistance KB carcinoma cells. Proc Natl Acad Sci USA 83: 4538–4542
18. Rowinsky EK, Burke PJ, Karp JE, Tucker RW, Ettinger DS, Donehower RC (1989) Phase 1 and pharmacodynamic study of taxol in refractory acute leukemias. Cancer Res 49: 4640–4647
19. Southern EM (1975) Detection of specific sequences among DNA fragments separated by gel electrophoresis. J Mol Biol 98: 503–517
20. Ueda K, Cardarelli C, Gottesman MM, Pastan I (1987) Expression of a full length cDNA for the human MDR1 gene confers resistance to colchicine, doxorubicin and vinblastine. Proc Natl Acad Sci USA 84: 3004–3008
21. White NJ, Looareesuwan S, Warrell DA, Warrell MJ, Bunnang D, Harinasuta T (1982) Quinine pharmacokinetics and toxicity in cerebral and uncomplicated falciparum malaria. Am J Med 73:564–568
22. Zamora PR, Pearce HL, Beck T (1988) Physical-chemical properties shared by compounds that modulate multidrug resistance in human leukemic cells. Mol Pharmacol 33: 454–462

Adhesion Molecules and Their Possible Influence on Immune Surveillance*

C.A. Schirren[1], H. Völpel[1], and S.C. Meuer[1]

Introduction

Besides facilitating cell to cell adhesion [8, 17, 20, 22], the molecular interactions between CD2 and its ligand CD58 (LFA-3), as well as between CD11a/18 (LFA-1) and CD54 (ICAM-1) have recently been recognized to participate in lymphocyte activation, recirculation, and effector function including cytolytic activity towards tumor cells [4, 5, 13–15, 18, 21, 24, 25] (Fig. 1). The involvement of CD54 and CD58 in cytolytic effector functions is obvious from blocking experiments employing monoclonal antibodies [12, 19, 23]. Besides the T cell receptor, CD2 is known to be capable of activating resting T lymphocytes and natural killer (NK) cells to express their functional repertoires, including cytotoxic activity [21]. In the case of NK cells, CD2 may represent the central triggering receptor whereas in T effector cells CD2 mediated signals appear to strongly synergize with the T cell receptor in amplifying immune responses [2, 14, 18, 21].

Ligands of CD2 such as sheep red blood cells (SRBC express the homologue of human CD58), recombinant, and natural human CD58 molecules, as well as particular monoclonal CD2 antibodies which mimic CD58 functions have been shown to exert triggering effects on T lymphocytes and NK cells [11, 14, 21, 22]. The availability of a sufficient number of corresponding CD58 molecules is strictly required to engage the CD2 dependent mode of T cell activation.

---

* This study is supported by a grant from the Tumorzentrum Heidelberg-Mannheim, C.A. Schirren is a recipient of a fellowship award from the Deutsche Forschungsgemeinschaft (DFG: Schi 284/1-1).

[1] Deutsches Krebsforschungszentrum, Abteilung Angewandte Immunologie, Im Neuenheimer Feld 280, W-6900 Heidelberg, FRG

G. Staehler S. Pomer (Eds.)
Basic and Clinical Research on Renal Cell Carcinoma

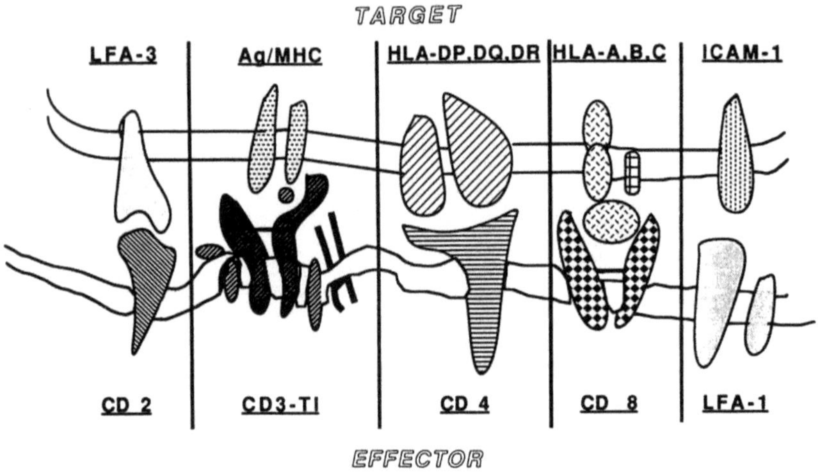

Fig. 1. Molecules involved in effector-target interaction and cell to cell adhesion

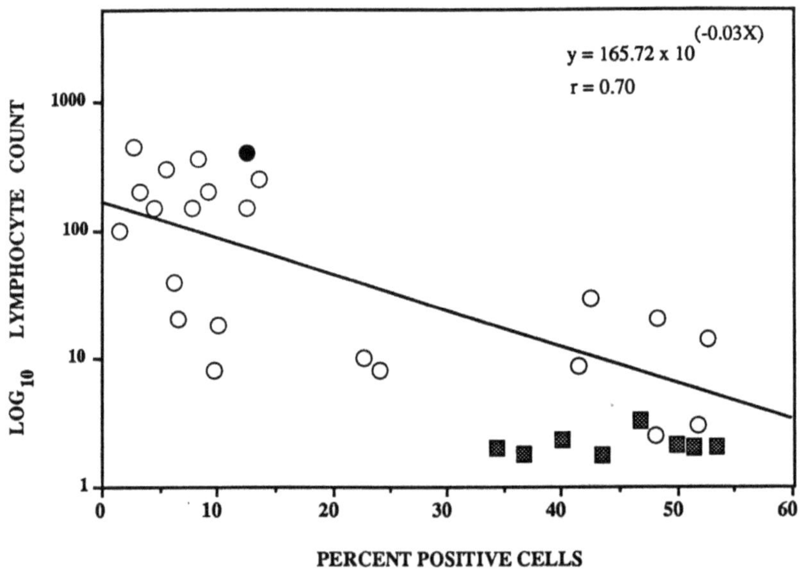

Fig. 2. Correlation between peripheral lymphocyte count and expression of CD54. LOG_{10} lymphocyte count is plotted against percent positive cells expressing CD54 molecules. Each *circle* represents one patient and the *boxes* CD54 expression of healthy donors. The *black point* marks the patient with T-PLL from which the effector cell line KEL-3 was established. There is a significant inverse correlation between the expression of CD54 on freshly recovered T leukemias and the lymphocyte count in the peripheral blood. For CD54: correlation coefficient $r = 0.7$

Conversely, blockade of CD58 binding to CD2 shuts off completely this alternative pathway of T cell triggering [11, 22].

On the surface of untransformed cells expression and densities of these glycoproteins vary considerably depending on the cellular differentiation state. For example, CD2 and CD58 expression increase by at least one order of magnitude following triggering of resting T lymphocytes to undergo clonal expansion. Moreover, upregulation of CD54 and CD58 expression has been observed in inflammatory sites and on endothelial cells following exposure to mediators [6, 7, 9, 16].

Conversely, downregulation of both molecules (CD54 and CD58) was recently shown to occur on EBV positive Burkitt lymphoma cell lines and has been suggested to facilitate tumor cell escape from virus specific T cell surveillance in vitro [3, 10]. Reduced expression of these molecules may protect tumor cells not only because of preventing cell to cell attachment but also due to not allowing efficient effector cell activation.

Results and Discussion

Correlation Between Expression of Adhesion Molecules and Accelerated Leukemic Disease

Expression of the cellular adhesion molecules CD58 (LFA-3), CD54 (ICAM-1) and CD11a (LFA-1) was investigated on a group of 23 freshly recovered human T cell leukemias (T acute lymphoblastic leukemia (T-ALL; four cases), T prolymphocytic leukemia (T-PLL; eleven cases), Sézary syndrome (SS; five cases), T chronic lymphocytic leukemia (T-CLL; three cases) [1] by indirect immunofluorescence employing an EPICS profile cytofluorograph. Figures 2 and 3 compare the expression of CD54 and CD58 on leukemic and nonleukemic peripheral blood lymphocytes (PBL) with the peripheral blood lymphocyte count in individual patients. As shown, there exists an inverse correlation between the degree of cell surface expression of CD54 and CD58 and the peripheral expansion of leukemic lymphoblasts in the patient's circulation. To confirm this observation, we performed a linear regression procedure with a level of significance alpha = 0.05. For CD54 the correlation coefficient is 0.7, and for CD58 the correlation coefficient is even higher, namely, 0.83 (Figs. 2, 3). Thus, in the presence of very high PBL counts there is a very low and sometimes undetectable surface expression of CD54 and CD58.

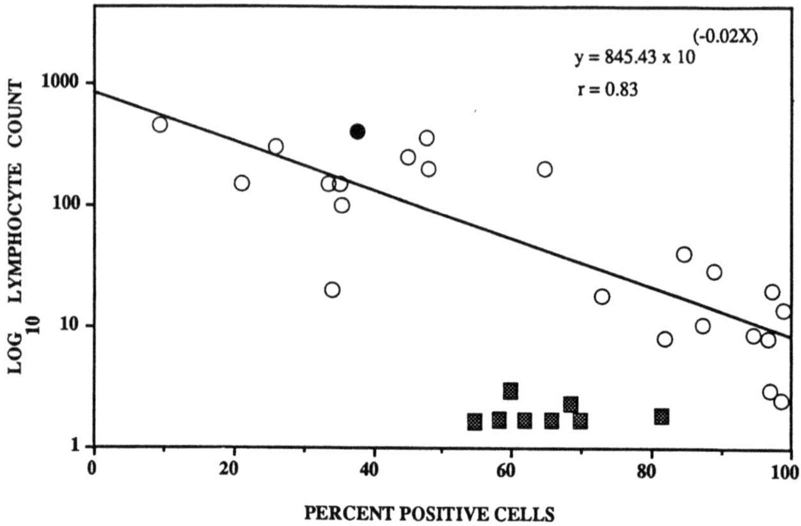

Fig. 3. Correlation between peripheral lymphocyte count and expression of CD58. LOG_{10} lymphocyte count is plotted against percent positive cells expressing CD58. Each *circle* represents one patient and the *boxes* CD58 expression of healthy donors. The *black point* marks the patient with T-PLL from which the effector cell line KEL-3 was established. There is a significant inverse correlation between the expression of CD58 on freshly recovered T leukemias and the lymphocyte count in the peripheral blood. For CD58: correlation coefficient $r = 0.83$

Figure 4 demonstrates surface expression of CD54 and CD58 on various cell populations of one representative patient (compare Fig. 2 and 3) as well as on resting and activated T cells from a healthy control individual. As demonstrated, malignant T lymphoblasts express very little CD54 and CD58 as compared to nontransformed blastoid T cells.

Our present analysis provides, for the first time, strong support for the view that indeed downregulation of CD54 and CD58 can exist in vivo and significantly correlates with accelerated leukemic disease (Figs. 2, 3). Although not shown, progression of disease in some patients was found to be accompanied by reduction of surface densities of CD54 and CD58. Moreover, in T cell lymphoma, a more localized disease, expression of adhesion molecules sometimes even exceeded the normal level. In contrast to CD54 and CD58 we found no such relation for CD11a/18 (LFA-1), CD2, major histocompatibility complex (MHC) class I and MHC class II (data not shown).

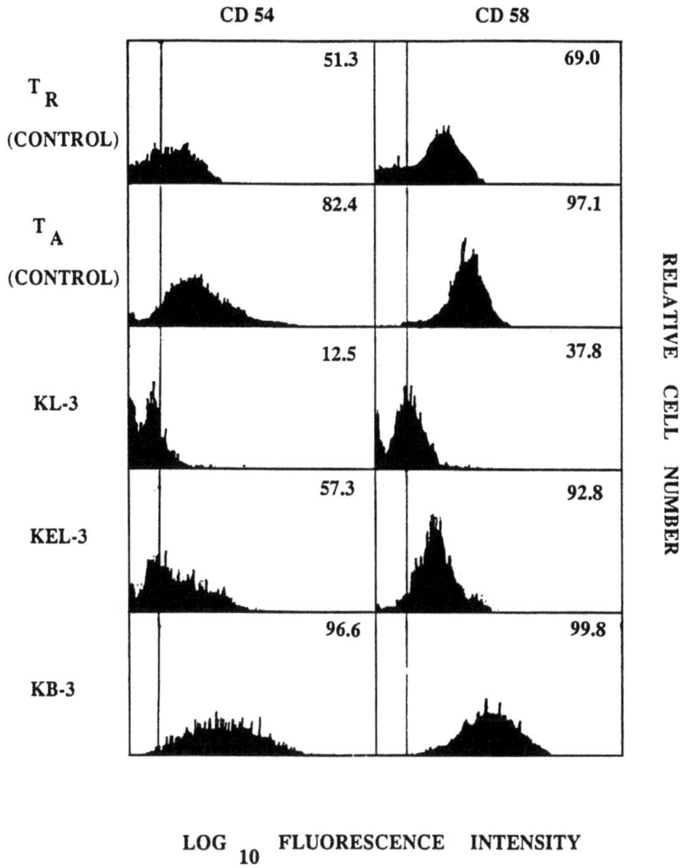

Fig. 4. Expression of CD54 and CD58 molecules on various cell types. T_R (control), resting T cells; T_A (control), activated T cell clone; *KL-3*, malignant T blasts from patient K with T-PLL; *KEL-3*, IL-2 dependent cytotoxic T effector line from patient K; *KB-3*, EBV transformed B-LCL from patient K. The position of the cursor was adjusted according to the negative control samples (<1% positive cells). The percentage of positive cells is represented by the *number* in each diagram

Malignant Lymphoblasts are not Capable of being Killed by Autologous Effector Cells

Given the inverse correlation between lymphocyte count and expression of CD54 and CD58 we now addressed the question whether down-regulation of adhesion molecules allows tumor cells to escape from

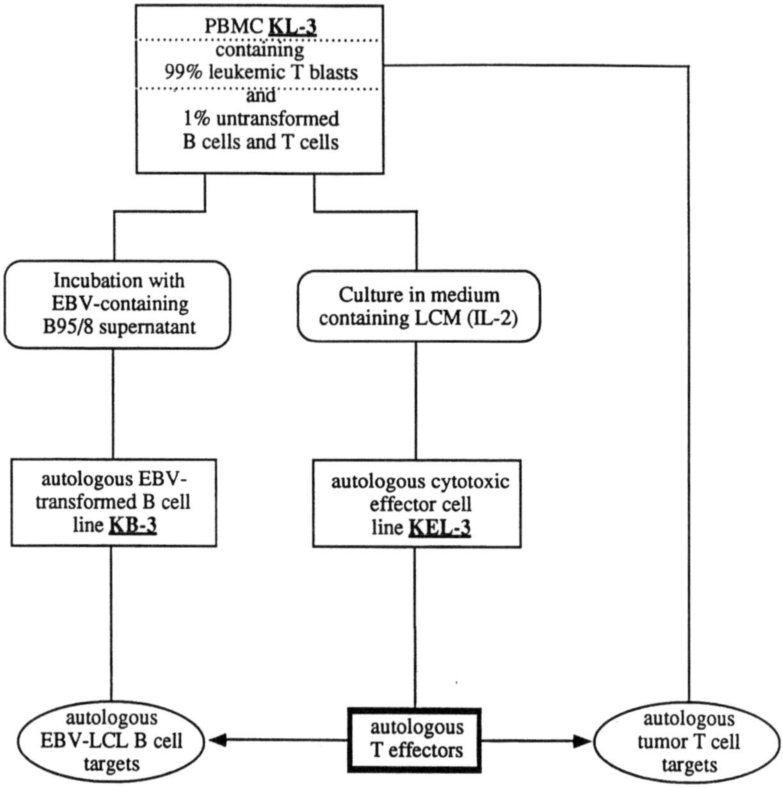

Fig. 5. Schematic diagram of establishing an autologous test system from one patient with a T-PLL

autologous killer cells. To this end we established an autologous in vitro test system from one patient which included an EBV transformed B lymphoblastoid cell line (B-LCL) KB-3, malignant lymphoblasts KL-3, and effector line KEL-3 (Figs. 4, 5).

In order to obtain nontransformed autologous effector lymphocytes which might be capable of eliminating leukemic T cell blasts, peripheral blood mononuclear cells of one patient (see Figs. 2, 3) were obtained and incubated with interleukin-2 in vitro (Fig. 5). The rationale of this approach was that those T lymphocytes which recognized tumor cells in the sample should acquire responsiveness to IL-2 and thus be selectively expanded in vitro. In fact, this experimental procedure led to the generation of a cell line, KEL-3 (compare Fig. 4), (phenotype: CD2 99%; CD3 90%; T-cell receptor alpha/beta 19%; T-cell receptor gamma/delta 70%; CD4 < 1.5%; CD8 30%;

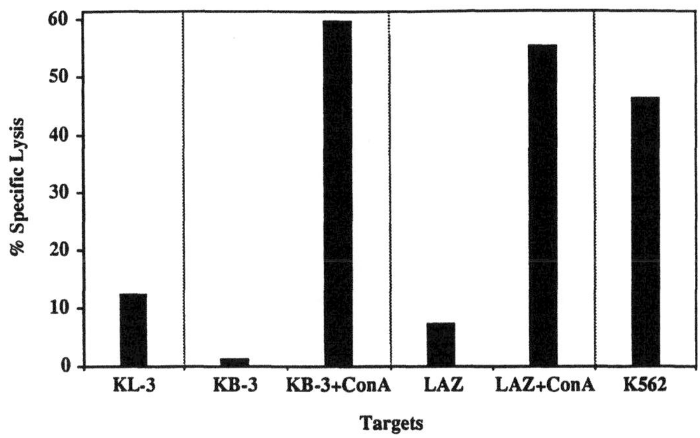

Fig. 6. Cytotoxic activity of the effector T cell line KEL-3. Lysis of autologous target KL-3, autologous EBV-LCL (KB-3), allogeneic EBV-LCL (LAZ 509), and erythroblastoid cell line K562 was measured in a 4-h standard ^{51}Cr release assay at an E to T ratio of 20/1. Con A was used at a final concentration of 10 μg/ml

CD16 24%; CD56 22%; MHC class I 100%; MHC class II 98%; CD54 57%; CD58 93%) which was capable of exerting strong lectin dependent cellular lysis towards autologous and unrelated target cells (Fig. 6). However, in the absence of lectin only background lytic activity could be observed towards the B-LCL KB-3 and LAZ 509 and, more important, the autologous T leukemia KL-3. In contrast, there was good killing activity towards the NK cell target K562.

Cytokines Modulate Expression of Adhesion Molecules in Tumor Cells

In a next set of experiments, we addressed the question whether upregulation of cell surface expression of CD54 and CD58 would render tumor cells more susceptible to autologous cell mediated lysis. To this end, leukemic blasts were incubated with interferon (IFN)-gamma (250 U/ml), tumor necrosis factor (TNF)-alpha (25 ng/ml), and IL-4 (100 U/ml), respectively, for 3 days.

As shown in Fig. 7, incubation in medium with fetal calf serum (FCS) for 3 days led to enhanced expression of CD54, and CD58, whereas practically no change was observed for CD11a. Addition of cytokines TNF-alpha (25 ng/ml), IFN-gamma (250 U/ml), IL-4 (100 U/ml) induced significant alterations in surface densities of CD54

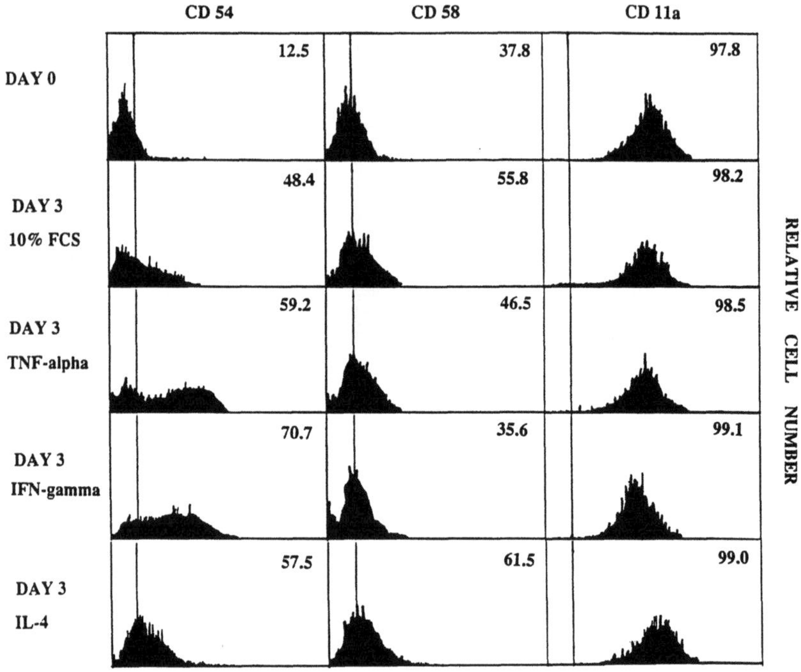

Fig. 7. Modulation of CD54, CD58 and CD11a expression by various cytokines on the malignant T blasts (KL-3). Concentrations of cytokines: TNF-alpha: 25 ng/ml; IFN-gamma: 250 U/ml; IL-4: 100 U/ml. The position of the cursor was adjusted according to the negative control samples (<1% positive cells). The percentage of positive cells is represented by the *number* in each diagram

and CD58. However, whereas CD54 expression was in general rather enhanced, CD58 molecules were found to become downregulated under these conditions. This differential influence on CD54 versus CD58 expression was particularly true for IFN-gamma. Note that the in vitro response of this particular leukemia sample is not representative for all cases investigated in our laboratory. Nevertheless, in almost each instance, one or the other mediator was capable of inducing changes in expression of the above mentioned adhesion molecules.

Modulation of Adhesion Molecules Renders Tumor Cells Susceptible for Autologous Effector Mechanisms

Given that recombinant mediators are capable of modulating expression of adhesion molecules, it was necessary to investigate whether

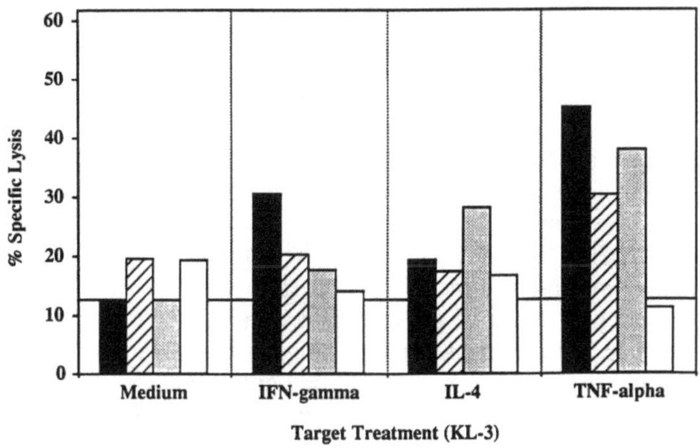

Fig. 8. Cytotoxic activity of the effector T cell line KEL-3 on lysis of cytokine treated autologous malignant blasts KL-3. T leukemic blasts KL-3 were incubated for 3 days with medium, IFN-gamma (250 U/ml), IL-4 (100 U/ml) or TNF-alpha (25 ng/ml), respectively. To inhibit cytolysis medium ■ or mAbs to CD11a (ELIIIG7) ▨, CD54 (WEHI-CAMI) ▩ or CD58 (TS 2/9) □ were added at a final dilution of 1:1000 (ascites in culture medium) to ^{51}Cr-labeled targets for 30 min at 4°C before addition of KEL-3

such alteration of the surface density of these glycoproteins would render tumor cells susceptible for autologous effector cells. As shown (Fig. 8), in the case of the TNF-alpha treated tumor cell sample, there was a strong lytic activity exerted by autologous cytotoxic lymphocytes. That this effector function involved CD54 and CD58 molecules is evident from the blocking experiments in which saturating concentrations of monoclonal antibodies directed at CD58 (and to a lesser extent CD54 and CD11a) reduced the level of killing down to the value that was obtained with untreated tumor cell targets (Fig. 6). Note that the autologous EBV transformed lymphoblastoid B cell line KB-3 was not lysed (Fig. 6) despite its strong expression of CD54 and CD58 (see Fig. 4), indicating a selectivity of the cell mediated immune response for autologous T leukemic blasts. Moreover, unlike leukemic T cell basts (KL-3) KB-3 cells were not lysed by KEL-3 even after incubation with recombinant mediators (not shown).

The fact that only the conditions induced by TNF-alpha allowed for tumor cell lysis stresses the point that both CD54 and CD58 are required for effector function. The moderate ability of autologous killer cells to affect KL-3 in the IFN-gamma treated sample may be explained by subthreshold expression of CD58, whereas the opposite may be the case for KL-3 cells that were exposed to IL-4, where "sufficient" expression of CD54 was not achieved. The nature of FCS related activities which in combination with recombinant cytokines were responsible for the observed effects is not known.

One additional conclusion results from the present experiments: the degree of tumor cell susceptibility to immunologic effector mechanisms may, to a large extent, depend on the degree of expression of cellular adhesion molecules by tumor cells. Our findings, therefore, stress the point that successful immunotherapy of malignant disease will depend on influencing both the immune response itself and the malignant tumor target. Thus, despite the fact that tumor specific lymphocytes could be generated in vivo by, for example, vaccination with purified tumor associated antigens or activation by lymphokines ex vivo, their potential of mediating antitumor effects in vivo may be limited due to a lack of expression of adhesion molecules on their respective targets.

The regulation of adhesion molecule expression by the tumor cells investigated here appears to be different than in untransformed cells since enhanced proliferation in the latter is usually accompanied by enhanced surface density of CD54 and CD58. In contrast here some of the most proliferating leukemias showed the lowest expression of CD54 and CD58. It should be noted that within inflammatory sites, virtually all cell types abundantly express CD54 and CD58, suggesting that mediators exist which are capable of inducing these adhesion molecules in vivo (own unpublished observations). Therefore, it will be necessary to examine whether particular mediators either alone or in combination synergize in their capacity of inducing CD54 and CD58 on T leukemia cells. This point is presently under investigation. Moreover, understanding the molecular regulation of cellular adhesion molecule expression on transformed and nontransformed cell types appears to be crucial for establishing a firm basis for immunotherapy. T leukemias as investigated here may provide powerful model systems which will help to understand these rules.

References

1. Bennett JM, Catovsky D, Daniel M-T, Flandrin G, Galton DAG, Gralnick HR, Sultan C (1989) The French-American-British (FAB) cooperative group. Proposals for the classification of chronic (mature) B and T lymphoid leukemias. J Clin Pathol 42: 567
2. Bierer BE, Peterson A, Gorga JC, Herrmann SH, Burakoff SJ (1988) Synergistic T cell activation via the physiological ligands for CD2 and the T cell receptor. J Exp Med 168: 1145
3. Billaud M, Calender A, Seigneurin J-M, Lenoir GM (1987) LFA-1, LFA-3, and ICAM-1 expression in Burkitt's lymphoma. Lancet ii: 1327

4. Carrera AC, Rincón M, Sánchez-Madrid F, López-Botet M, de Landazuri MO (1988) Triggering of co-mitogenic signals in T cell proliferation by anti-LFA-1 (CD18, CD11a), LFA-3, and CD7 monoclonal antibodies. J Immunol 141: 1919
5. Clayberger C, Wright R, Medeiros LJ et al. (1987) Absence of cell surface LFA-1 as a mechanism of escape from immunosurveillance. Lancet ii: 533
6. Cosimi AB, Conti D, Delmonico FL et al. (1990) In vivo effects of monoclonal antibody to ICAM-1 (CD54) in non-human primates with renal allografts. J Immunol 144: 4604
7. Dustin ML, Springer TA (1989) T-cell receptor cross-linking transiently stimulates adhesiveness through LFA-1. Nature 341: 619
8. Dustin ML, Singer KH, Tuck DT, Springer TA (1988) Adhesion of lymphoblasts to epidermal keratinocytes is regulated by Interferon-gamma and is mediated by intercellular adhesion molecule 1 (ICAM-1). J Exp Med 167: 1323
9. Faull RJ, Russ GR (1989) Tubular expression of intercellular adhesion molecule-1 during renal allograft rejection. Transplantation 48: 226
10. Gregory CD, Murray RJ, Edwards CF, Rickinson AB (1988) Downregulation of cell adhesion molecules LFA-3 and ICAM-1 in Epstein-Barr virus-positive Burkitt's lymphoma underlies tumor cell escape from virus-specific T cell surveillance. J Exp Med 167: 1811
11. Hünig T, Tiefenthaler G, Meyer zum Büschenfelde K-H, Meuer SC (1987) Alternative pathway activation of T cells by binding of CD2 to its cell-surface ligand. Nature 326: 298
12. Krensky AM, Sanchez-Madrid F, Robbins E, Nagy JA, Springer TA, Burakoff SJ (1983) The functional significance, distribution, and structure of LFA-1, LFA-2, and LFA-3: Cell surface antigens associated with CTL-target interactions. J Immunol 131: 611
13. Makgoba MW, Sanders ME, Ginther Luce GE, Gugel EA, Dustin ML, Springer TA, Shaw S (1988) Functional evidence that intercellular adhesion molecule-1 (ICAM-1) is a ligand for LFA-1-dependent adhesion in T cell-mediated cytotoxicity. Eur J Immunol 18: 637
14. Meuer SC, Hussey RE, Fabbi M, et al. (1984) An alternative pathway of T cell activation: A functional role of the 50 kD T11 sheep erythrocyte receptor protein. Cell 36: 897
15. Pardi R, Bender JR, Dettori C, Giannazza E, Engleman EG (1989) Heterogenous distribution and transmembrane signaling properties of lymphocyte function-associated antigen (LFA-1) in human lymphocyte subsets. J Immunol 143: 3157
16. Patarroyo M, Makgoba MW (1989) Leukocyte adhesion to cells in immune and inflammatory responses. Lancet ii: 1139
17. Rothlein R, Dustin ML, Marlin SD, Springer TA (1986) A human intercellular adhesion molecule (ICAM-1) distinct from LFA-1. J Immunol 137: 1270
18. Schraven B, Roux M, Hutmacher B, Meuer SC (1989) Triggering of the alternative pathway of human T cell activation involves members of the T 200 family of glycoproteins. Eur J Immunol 19: 397
19. Shaw S, Ginther Luce GE (1987) The lymphocyte function-associated antigen (LFA)-1 and CD2/LFA-3 pathways of antigen-independent human T cell adhesion. J Immunol 139: 1037

20. Shaw S, Ginther Luce GE, Quinones R, Grass RE, Springer TA, Sanders ME (1986) Two antigen-independent adhesion pathways used by human cytotoxic T-cell clones. Nature 323: 262
21. Siliciano RF, Pratt JC, Schmidt RE, Ritz J, Reinherz EL (1985) Activation of cytolytic T lymphocyte and natural killer cell function through the T11 sheep erythrocyte binding protein. Nature 317: 428
22. Tiefenthaler G, Hünig T, Dustin ML, Springer TA, Meuer SC (1987) Purified lymphocyte function-associated antigen-3 and T11 target structure are active in CD2-mediated T cell stimulation. Eur J Immunol 17: 1847
23. Ware CF, Sanchez-Madrid F, Krensky AM, Burakoff SJ, Strominger JL, Springer TA (1983) Human lymphocyte function associated antigen-1 (LFA-1): Identification of multiple antigenic epitopes and their relationship to CTL-mediated cytotoxocity. J Immunol 131: 1182
24. van Seventer GA, Shimizu Y, Horgan KJ, Shaw S (1990) The LFA-1 ligand ICAM-1 provides an important costimulatory signal for T cell receptor-mediated activation of resting T cells. J Immunol 144: 4579
25. van Noesel C, Miedema F, Brouwer M, de Rie MA, Aarden LA, van Lier RAW (1988) Regulatory properties of LFA-1 alpha and beta chains in human T-lymphocyte activation. Nature 333: 850

Immunobiology of Renal Cell Carcinoma

Anti-Proliferative and Anti-Tumor Effect of α-Interferon in Renal Cell Carcinoma: Correlation with the Expression of a Kidney Associated Differentiation Glycoprotein

N.H. Bander[1,2], G. Gastl[1,2], D.M. Nanus[3,4], L.M. Pfeffer[5], C.L. Finstad[2], and A.P. Albino[3]

Introduction

Approximately 20000 cases of renal cell carcinoma (RCC) are diagnosed annually in the US. About 25% of these patients have overt metastatic disease at the time of presentation. The median duration of survival in these patients have been reported to be approximately 10 months. Among the rest of the patients with cancers apparently localized to the kidney, the sole effective therapy is surgical excision of the cancer, typically by a radical nephrectomy. About one third of these patients with apparently localized disease (i.e., 25% of the total) will later manifest metastatic disease and ultimately succumb to the cancer. The annual mortality rate for renal cancer in the US is approximately 10000.

Metastatic renal cancer has proven to be resistant to both hormonal and nonhormonal chemotherapeutic agents [12]. Immunotherapeutic strategies seem to be demonstrating greater promise, however. Currently, the two most active agents are interleukin-2 (IL-2) and alpha-interferon (IFN). IL-2, with or without lymphokine activated killer cells, has produced response rates in the range of 0%–35% [1, 6, 7, 10]. The treatment is intense, and the toxicity is substantial. Trials of IFN have produced objective response rates of 5%–29% [2, 3, 5, 8, 11] with less side effects than seen in IL-2 trials. There has been no randomized trial comparing response rates of these

[1] Division of Urology, New York Hospital-Cornell Medical Center, 525 East 68th Street, New York, NY 10021, USA
[2] Laboratory of Human Cancer Immunology; [3] Laboratory of Mammalian Cell Transformation; [4] Division of Solid Tumor Oncology, Memorial Sloan-Kettering Cancer Center, 1275 York Avenue, New York, NY, USA
[5] Rockefeller University Hospital, New York, NY, USA

G. Staehler S. Pomer (Eds.)
Basic and Clinical Research on Renal Cell Carcinoma

two modalities in patients with renal cancer. Nevertheless, the reported response rates of IL-2 and IFN based studies are quite comparable despite the generally better performance status, lower tumor burden, and more favorable distribution of metastatic sites (pulmonary lesions respond better than bone) of the patients entering the IL-2 based studies. The lower morbidity of IFN and its general availability make IFN a very reasonable choice relative to IL-2.

IFN therapy, however, is not without problems of its own. It is expensive, and it is not without side effects. The problems of expense and toxicity are compounded by the long interval required to demonstrate response (median: 3 months [5]) plus the fact that only about 1 in 5 patients who endure these problems will derive an objective response.

Results and Discussion

In the course of studies characterizing human renal cancer cell lines for cell surface antigen expression and biologic properties (e.g., growth factor production, growth on soft agar, tumorigenicity in nude mice, etc.), we noted an antiproliferative and antitumor response in a subset of established human renal cancer cell lines when incubated with recombinant IFN-α (r-met-HuIFN-Conl, a consensus analogue of the most frequent amino acid residues known to occur in subspecies of IFN-α; provided by Amgen, Inc.). This appeared to be a direct effect, occurring in the absence of any immune effector cells. Furthermore, the observed antitumor effect was noted at concentrations of IFN which could be achieved in vivo. When both the IFN sensitive and resistant cell lines were molecularly phenotyped with six monoclonal antibodies (mAbs) defining kidney-restricted differentiation antigens (Table 1), the binding pattern of one mAb (F33) demonstrated a 95% concordance with response to IFN (Table 2).

mAb F33 detects a 160000-kDa glycoprotein expressed by normal glomerular and proximal tubular epithelial cells and by a subset of renal cancers in vivo and in vitro. All nine gp160+ cell lines tested which expressed gp160 (gp160+) were resistant to the antiproliferative effect of IFN, while eight of nine gp160− cell lines were IFN sensitive. This observation becomes even more provocative when juxtaposed to another study of about 200 renal cancer specimens in which the incidence of gp160− renal cancers (the putative IFN sensitive phenotype) accounted for approximately 20% of all renal cancers (Bander, Finstad, Cordon-Cardo, unpublished observations), or approximately the incidence of responses seen in clinical trials of IFN.

Table 1. Monoclonal antibodies

Designation (Ig subclass)	Mr of antigen	Site of expression
mAbF33 (γ1)	160000	G, PT
mAbS22 (γ1)	115000	RC only
mAbS23 (γ1)	120000	PT, LH
mAbT43 (γ1)	85000	PT_c
mAbF23 (γ2a)	140000	PT
mAbF31 (μ)	glycolipid	PT_s

G, Glomerulus; *PT*, proximal tubule; *LH*, loop of Henle; *RC*, renal cancer; PT_c, proximal tubule – convoluted; PT_s, proximal tubule – straight

Table 2. Expression of kidney differentiation antigens and interferon-α effect

	Antibodies						
Cell lines	S22	S23	T43	F23	F31	F33	IFN-α effect[1]
PT1	○	●	●	●	○	●	R
PT2	○	●	●	●	○	●	R
SK-RC-1	●	●	●	●	○	●	R
SK-RC-4	●	●	○	○	○	●	R
SK-RC-12		●	●	○	○	●	R
SK-RC-26	○	●	●	○	○	●	R
SK-RC-28	○	●	●	○	○	●	R
SK-RC-38		●	●	●	●	●	R
SK-RC-45	●	●	●	●	○	●	R
SK-RC-35		●	●	○	○	○	R
SK-RC-2	●	○	●	●	○	○	S
SK-RC-17		●	●	●	●	○	S
SK-RC-29	○	●	●	●	○	○	S
SK-RC-39		●	●	●	○	○	S
SK-RC-41		●	●	○	○	○	S
SK-RC-42	○	●	●	●	○	○	S
SK-RC-44		●	●	○	●	○	S
SK-RC-49		●	●	●	●	○	S

[1] IFN-α effect determined by growth inhibition assays (see ref. [4]). (*S*) indicates a >50% inhibition of cell growth as compared to untreated control cultures at an IFN-α concentration less than 1000 units/ml (except for SK-RC-29, where 50% inhibition occurred at 3000 units/ml). (*R*) indicates <20% inhibition of cell growth as compared to untreated control cultures at an IFN-α concentration up to 3000 units/ml. ●, strong reactivity; ○, weak reactivity; ○, no reactivity by cell binding assays

We wanted to do a retrospective study of gp160 expression in patients previously entered in clinical trials of IFN to attempt to validate the in vitro findings. Unfortunately, this was not feasible as gp160 expression cannot be determined on routinely processed (i.e., formaldehyde fixed, paraffin embedded) tissue. Like most mAbs to protein antigens, immunopathological determination requires analysis on frozen sections. We, therefore, elected to study a nude mouse-human renal cancer xenograft model to determine whether systemic in vivo administration of IFN would yield results similar to those we had observed in vitro. Seven established human renal cancer cell lines (two gp160+, five gp160−) known to grow in nude mice were selected. Harvested cells from each line were injected subcutaneously into groups of 8–10 mice. Half of each group was treated with 1 million units IFN intraperitoneally three times weekly, starting on the day of tumor inoculation. The remaining mice in each group served as untreated controls. Mice were monitored for tumor formation, which was defined as the time of initial presentation of a subcutaneous nodule >/= 2 mm which continued to enlarge. The results are shown in Table 3. All of the untreated mice developed tumors regardless of gp160 expression. Among the IFN treated groups, mice inoculated with gp160+ cell lines developed tumors just like their untreated counterparts; mice inoculated with gp160− tumors demonstrated significant delay or prevention of tumor take. The data was, therefore, entirely consistent with the in vitro data. We investigated the possi-

Table 3. Antiproliferative effect of inteferon-α on renal cancer xenografts

Cell line	gp160 expression	Median days to tumor formation[a] −IFN-α	Median days to tumor formation[a] +IFN-α[b]
SK-RC-01	+	14	15
SK-RC-45	+	10	10
SK-RC-17	−	6	>77
SK-RC-39	−	30	>73
SK-RC-42	−	40	NTF
SK-RC-44	−	7	NTF
SK-RC-49	−	5	NTF

NTF, No tumor formation

[a] Tumor formation assessed as the initial presentation of a subcutaneous nodule >2 mm which continued to enlarge.

[b] IFN-α is treatment with 1 million units of recombinant DNA derived α-IFN-CON 1 intraperitoneally on a M-W-F schedule (see ref. [4])

bility that gp160 is related to the multi-drug resistance (*mdr*) gene product (p170) because of their similar molecular weight, *mdr*'s known expression in renal tissue, and the role of *mdr* in resistance to chemotherapeutic agents. Our analysis indicates that p170 is different from gp160. Immunohistochemical analysis demonstrates different patterns of expression of these two molecules. For example, in normal kidney, gp160 is expressed by both glomerular and proximal tubular cells while p170 expression is limited to the proximal tubule. In addition, p170 is expressed by the adrenal, pancreas, and portions of the intestine while gp160 is not expressed by any of these tissues [9]. In addition, RCC cell lines in vitro do not co-phenotype with mAbs to gp160 and p170.

If gp160 does mediate IFN resistance, its effect is likely limited to renal cancer as gp160 is a highly restricted renal differentiation antigen and is not expressed by other normal tissues or cancers (with the exception that some sarcomas appear to be gp160+).

It is not yet clear whether gp160 directly mediates IFN resistance or if gp160 merely fortuitously co-types with another gene product which is responsible for IFN resistance. However, we have found that there is a correlation between the apparent level of cell surface gp160 expression and IFN resistance. Of seven RCC lines which were gp160− by cell binding assay and by immunoprecipitation, all had an IC_{50} dose of under 1000 U/ml. Cell lines with higher levels of expression required variously higher concentrations of IFN to reach the IC_{50}. These higher dose levels exceed that attainable in vivo.

We attempted to block IFN resistance in gp160+ RCC lines in vitro using mAbs to gp160. We could not demonstrate any change in resistance. This could indicate that gp160 does not directly mediate the resistance or that the mAbs utilized do not block the active site.

Summary

In conclusion, we have observed an antiproliferative or antitumor effect among a subset of human renal cancers when incubated with IFN in vitro or when grown in an animal model and systemically treated with IFN. In neither setting does the response require the presence of immune effector cells. In 95% of the RCC lines tested (17 of 18), the response to IFN correlates with the expression of a kidney-restricted differentiation antigen, gp160. The sensitive phenotype (gp160−) occurs in approximately 20% of patients with real cancer – approximately the response rate reported in numerous clinical trials.

Recently, a prospective trial has begun to test the hypothesis that the gp160 phenotype is predictive of IFN response in patients. If confirmed, such a finding would be of obvious practical benefit.

Lastly, it is not currently known if gp160 directly mediates IFN resistance or merely co-types with another gene product responsible for the phenomenon. Nor is the function of gp160 known. We are currently endeavoring to clone the gene to answer these questions. If gp160 does mediate the resistance, it is tempting to contemplate the possibility of blocking its function. This could theoretically lead to higher response rates in patients with RCC treated with IFN.

References

1. Abrams JS, Rayner AA, Wiernik PH, et al. (1990) High-dose recombinant interleukin-2 alone: A regimen with limited activity in the treatment of advanced renal cell carcinoma. J Natl Cancer Inst 82: 1202–1206
2. Fosså SD, De Garis ST, Heier MS, et al. (1986) Recombinant interferon alfa-2a with or without vinblastine in metastatic renal cell carcinoma. Cancer 57: 1700–1704
3. Krown SE (1987) Interferon treatment of renal cell carcinoma – Current status and future prospects. Cancer 59: 647–651
4. Nanus DM, Pfeffer LM, Bander NH, et al. (1990) Antiproliferative and antitumor effects of -Interferon in renal cell carcinomas: Correlation with the expression of a kidney-associated differentiation glycoprotein. Cancer Res 50: 4190–4194
5. Neidhart JA (1986) Interferon therapy for the treatment of renal cancer. Cancer 57: 1696–1699
6. Parkinson DR, Fisher RI, Rayner AA, et al. (1990) Therapy of renal cell carcinoma with interleukin-2 and lymphokine-activated killer cells: Phase II experience with a hybrid bolus and continuous infusion interleukin-2 regimen. J Clin Oncol 8: 1630–1636
7. Rosenberg SA, Lotze MT, Muul LM, et al. (1987) A progress report on the treatment of 157 patients with advanced cancer using lymphokine-activated killer cells and interleukin-2 or high-dose interleukin-2 alone. N Engl J Med 316: 889
8. Sarna G, Figlin R, de Kernion J (1987) Interferon in renal cell carcinoma – The UCLA experience. Cancer 59: 610–612
9. Thiebaut F, Tsuruo T, Hamada H, et al. (1987) □ Proc Natl Acad Sci USA 84: 7735–7738
10. Wang JCL, Walle A, Novogrodsky A, et al. (1989) A phase II clinical trial of adoptive immunotherapy for advanced renal cell carcinoma using mitogen-activated autologous leukocytes and continuous infusion interleukin-2. J Clin Oncol 7: 1885–1891
11. Umeda T, Niijima T (1986) Phase II study of alpha interferon on renal cell carcinoma – Summary of three collaborative trials. Cancer 58: 1231–1235
12. Yagoda A, Bander NH (1989) Failure of cytotoxic chemotherapy, 1983–1988, and the emerging role of monoclonal antibodies for renal cancer. Urol Int 44: 338–345

Prediction of Cytokine-Therapy on Basis of Class-I and Class-II MHC Antigen Induction

A.J.M.C. Beniers, W.P. Peelen, F.M.J. Debruyne, and J.A. Schalken[1]

Introduction

Cytokine therapy has proven to be effective in approximately 15% of the patients with metastatic renal cell carcinoma (RCC). In the further implementation of this still experimental therapeutic modality, two questions are considered relevant, i.e., how can the optimal cytokine treatment combination and dosage be determined, and are there markers predicting a response. Recent findings indicate that the optimal doses can vary for individual patients [2]. Moreover, insight into the best combination of cytokines is not yet available. In the identification of patients that respond to immunotherapy, both host mediated effects as well as tumor cell characteristics should be considered. In this study special emphasis was given to the role of histocompatibility antigens as a predictor for response. These molecules play an important role in both the presentation of autologous and or heterologous antigens to the immune system and result in eventual binding and elimination. Furthermore, it has been recognized that these molecules can be induced by several cytokines. In a previous study in which we studied the cytokine sensitivity of eight human RCC xenografts in a nude mouse model we found a variable response to the treatment with interferon-alpha, – gamme and tumor necrosis factor (TNF) [4]. In the same model we evaluated the level of expression of histocompatibility leucocyte antigens (HLA) and the modulation by cytokines. The nude mouse model does not permit conclusions regarding the functional role of these molecules in an eventual host mediated response induced by immunotherapy; however, the expression and inducibility of HLA class-I and class-II

[1] Urologic Research Laboratory, Department of Urology, University Hospital Nijmegen, P.O. Box 9101, 6500 HB Nijmegen, The Netherlands

G. Staehler S. Pomer (Eds.)
Basic and Clinical Research on Renal Cell Carcinoma

molecules can be correlated with the nonimmune mediated antitumor response.

Material and Methods

Renal Cell Carcinoma Xenografts

The NC-65 renal tumor xenograft [6] was kindley provided by Dr. J.C. Romijn from the Department of Urology, Erasmus University, Rotterdam, The Netherlands. All NU lines were established in our own laboratory [5]. Tumor stage of the primary tumors varied between T2 and T4.

Mice

Six-week-old male or female BalbC nu/nu mice (Bomholtgård, Ry, Denmark) were used. Prior to the start of the experiments, the animals were adjusted to the experimental environment for 2 weeks.

Cytokines

Human interferon (IFN)-alpha, IFN-gamma and TNF-alpha, kindly supplied by Boehringer Ingelheim, Alkmaar, The Netherlands, were produced in *Escherichia coli* by recombinant DNA technology. The specific activity of IFN-alpha and IFN-gamma was $3.2 \times 10E8$ units/mg protein and $2 \times 10E7$ units/mg, respectively. The specific activity of TNF-alpha determined in the presence of actinomycin-D was $6 \times 10E7$ units/mg (the L-929 cytotoxicity assay). The cytokines were dissolved in the accessory dissolvent and diluted with unsupplemented RPMI medium (Gibco, Paisley, UK) After dilution, the drugs were stored in 1.2 ml aliquotes at −80°C until use.

Treatment of Tumor Bearing Mice

Each treatment group consisted of five mice. Both male and female mice were used because previous experiments showed no differences in growth characteristics. Six-week-old mice were subcutaneously implanted with tumour tissue 1–2 mm^3 in size in the right flank.

Treatment groups were randomized before start of therapy and treatment started when tumors had grown to a volume of about 65 mm^3 (10–14 days after implantation), or 24–48 h after implantation of the tumor tissue. The animals were treated by subcutaneous administration peritumorally three or five times a week for 6 weeks. Each administration amounted to a total volume of 200 µl. Interferons (150 or 1500 U/g = 0.5 or 5.0 and 8.0 or 80.0 ng/g for alpha-IFN and gamma-IFN, respectively) were administered three times a week and TNF (30 000 U/g = 500 ng/g) was administered three or five times a week. Control mice were treated with the unsupplemented RPMI three times a week.

Three to six hours after the last peritumoral injection, the mice were killed by cervical dislocation of the spinal tract. The tumors were taken out and immediately snap frozen and stored in liquid nitrogen for immunohistochemical purposes or at −80 °C for mRNA expression studies of northern analyses.

Immunohistochemistry

Four cryostat sections of tumour tissue µm thick were stained by means of the direct immunoperoxidase technique using 3-3′diaminobenzidine (DAB) and hydrogen peroxide as substrates. Monoclonal antibodies used were W.6.32 for HLA-A,B,C (Class I) expression [3] and B8.11.2 for HLA-DR (Class II) expression [7].

RNA Isolation and Northern Blot Analyses

Total RNA from tumors was isolated using the lithium chloride/urea procedure as described by Auffray and Rougeon [1]. For northern blot analyses 10 µg of total RNA was glyoxylated, size fractioned on 1% agarose gels and transferred to Hybond-N+ nylon membrane (Amersham). Hybridization was carried out with the radioactively labelled plasmids pDP001 and DR alpha 120 (American Type Culture Collection) containing the human genes for HLA-B7 (HLA Class I) and HLA-DRA1 (HLA-DR Class II alpha chain), respectively [9, 10].

To quantitate the expression levels of HLA antigens in the different tumor lines, autoradiographs were scanned with an LKB Ultroscan XL enhanced laser densitometer connected to an Ultroscan XL 2000 integrator for integration of the data. Values of the untreated control groups were arbitrarily given the value 1.

Short-term In Vitro Culture Test

Tumor samples from the tumor lines or primary tumors were minced with scissors and after washing in unsupplemented RPMI-1640 culture medium, tumor sections of about 1 mm^3 were incubated in supplemented RPMI-1640 medium for 3 days into a 75-cm^2 tissue culture flask. Attached cells were checked for morphological characteristics. After typsinizing, the cells were incubated further for one night on glass slides in supplemented RPMI-1640 medium. Single doses of alpha- or gamma-IFN were added next in concentrations of 0.5 or 5 ng/ml. After 3 days, the dishes were washed in phosphate-buffered saline (PBS) and HLA antigen expression was tested by means of the direct immunoperoxidase assay.

Results

The results of the immunohistochemical and the northern analyses are shown in Figs. 1 and 2. Generally, the qualitative impression regarding HLA class I and II expression obtained by immunohistochemical studies corroborated the semi-quantitative determination of the HLA class I and II expression by northern analyses. Only in cases of the immunohistochemical analyses of the class II antigens, however, was additional information obtained by this technique, i.e. the fraction of positive cells increased.

HLA Class I Expression on Untreated and Cytokine Treated Renal Tumor Xenografts

Both the basal expression level and the extent of modulation after therapy varied considerably amongst the xenografts. A comparative analysis of the basal HLA class I expression in the RCC xenografts revealed that two of the lines, NU-3 and NU-20, show a very low basal class I expression, whereas the NU-5 and NU-22 lines show a very high basal class I expression (Table 1).

Upon cytokine treatment of NU-3 and NU-20 bearing mice, class I expression was induced only to a minor extent (less than threefold, Fig. 2) and highest modulation of class I expression is seen in the alpha-IFN 5.0/TNF 500 ng/g treated groups. In general, higher class I expression is found for the groups treated with the high IFN dose and, although the differences are very small, HLA class-I expression is

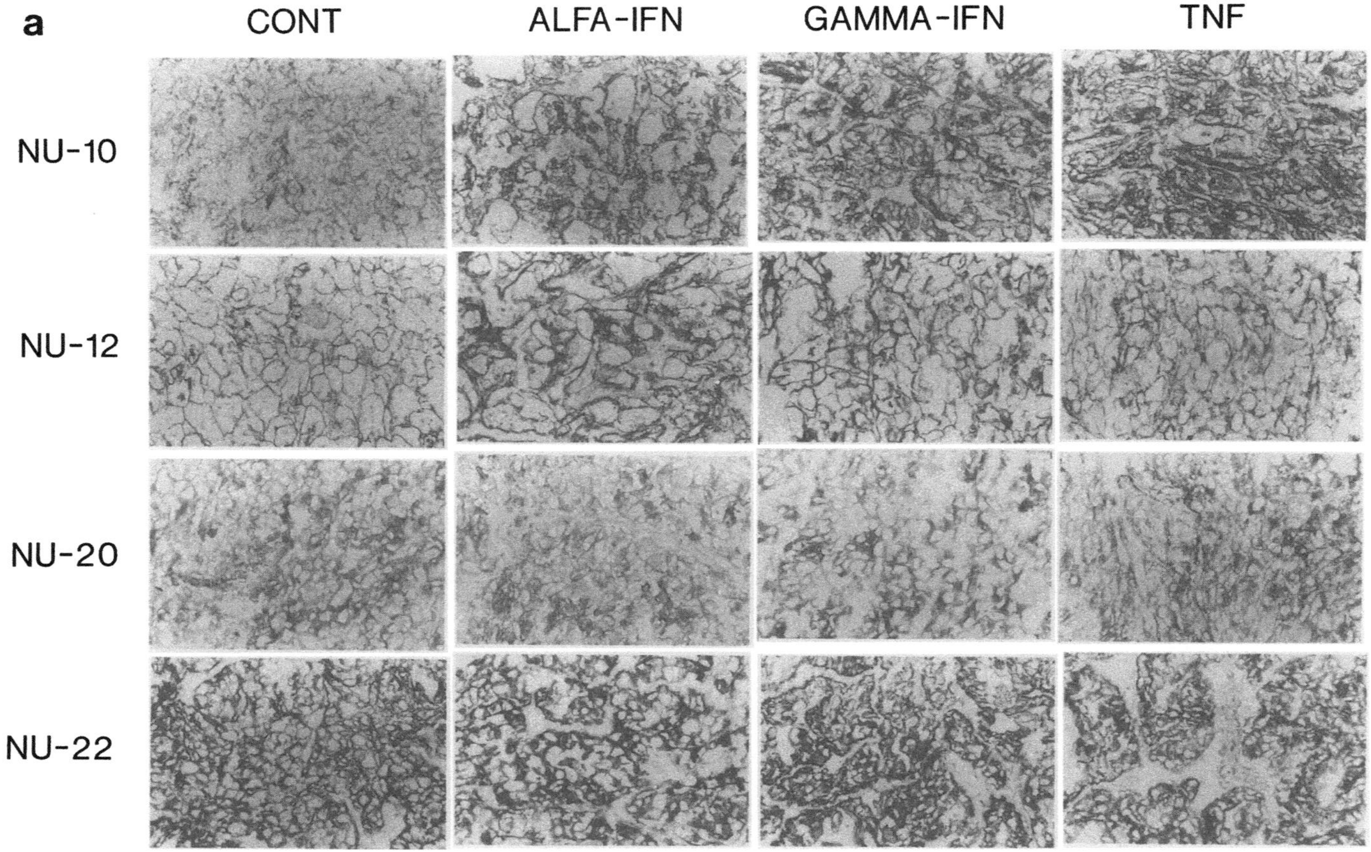

Fig. 1a, b. Immunohistochemical analysis of HLA class I (**a**) and HLA class II (**b**) antigens on RCC xenografts. The monoclonal antibodies used were W6.32 (class I) and B8.11.2 (class II) in a DAB peroxidase assay. Tumor lines: *NU-10*; *NU-12*; *NU-20*; *NU-22*; *CONT*, untreated control; *alfa-IFN*, alpha-IFN treated; *gamma-IFN*, gamma-IFN treated; *TNF*, TNF treated

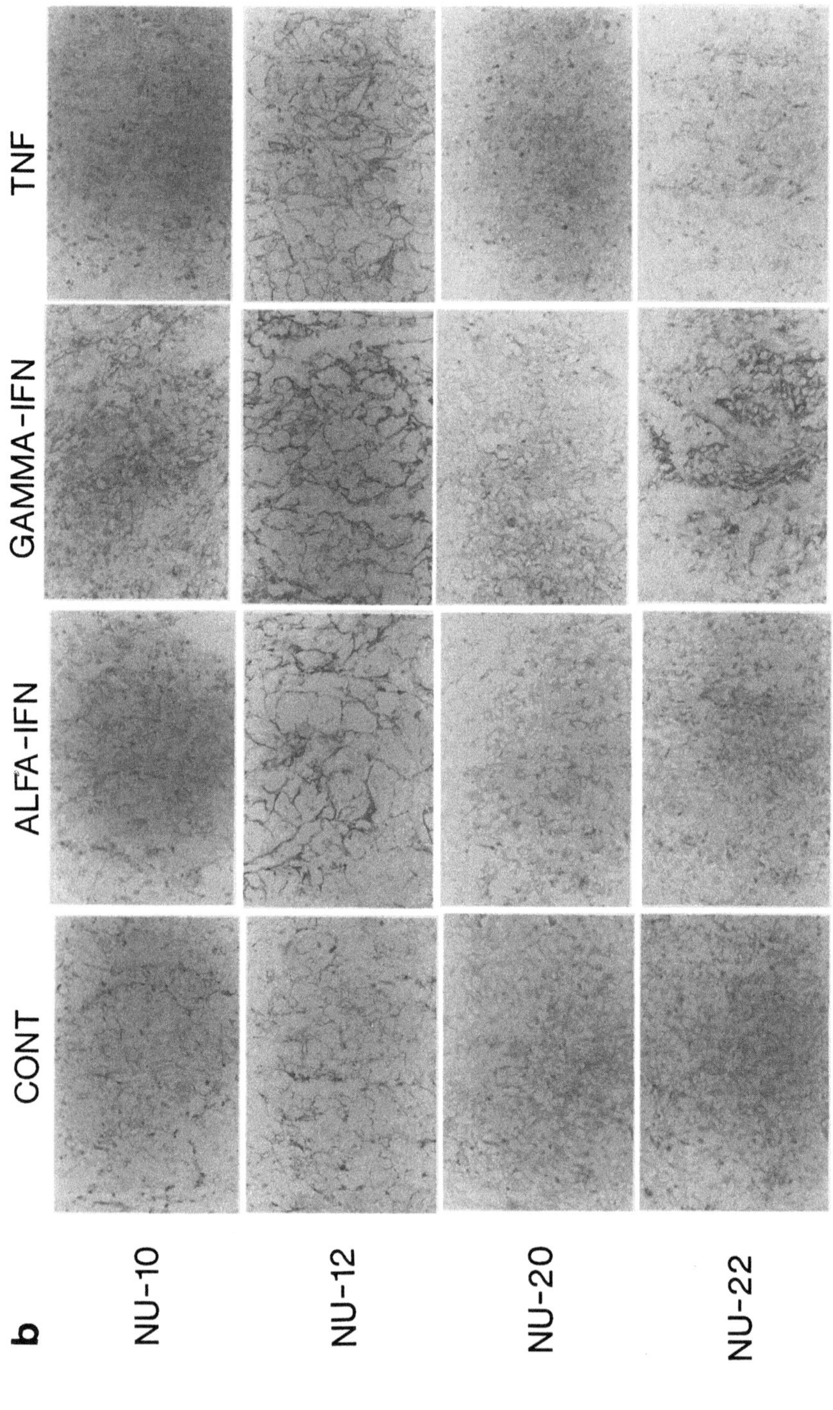
b
TNF
GAMMA-IFN
ALFA-IFN
CONT
NU-10
NU-12
NU-20
NU-22

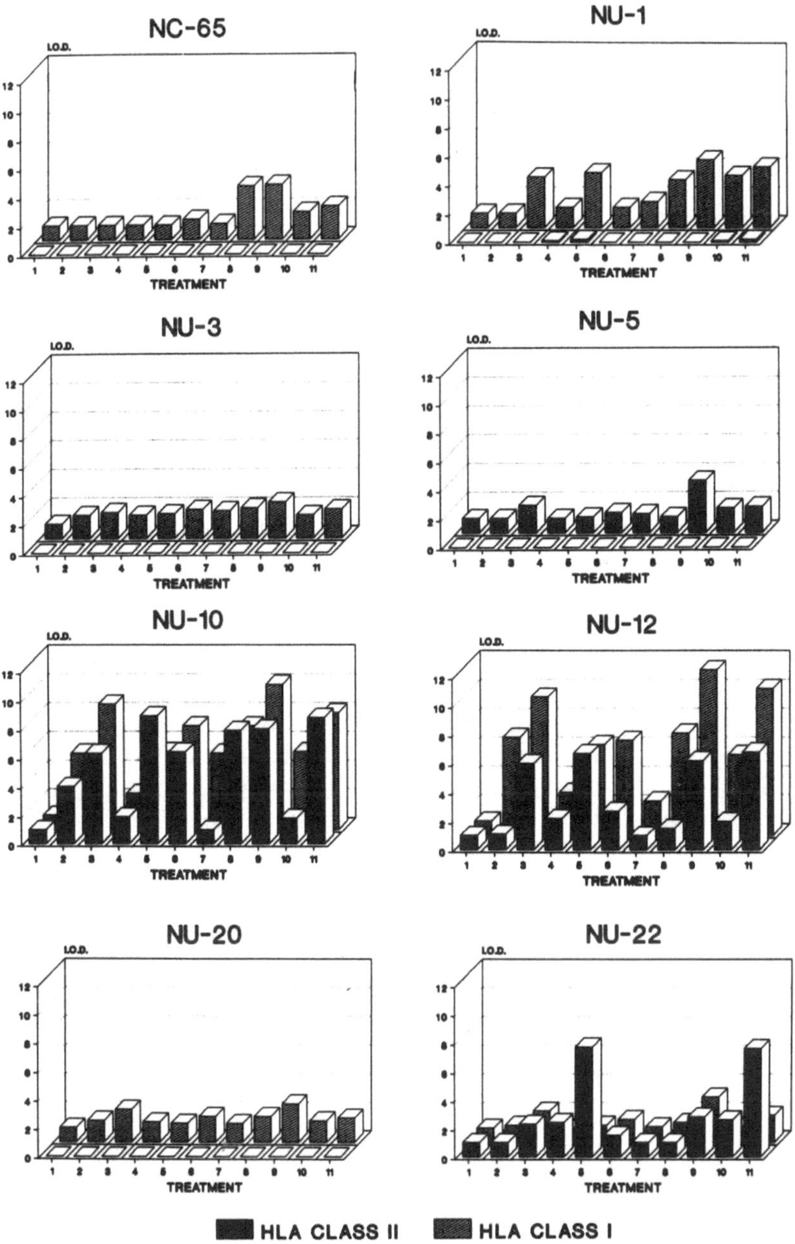

Fig. 2. Relative integrated optical densities on northern blot autoradiograms of HLA class I and class II expression on eight different xenografts subcutaneously growing in BalbC nu/nu mice treated with different combinations of cytokines. Treatments were as follows: *1*, control; *2*, alpha-IFN 0.5; *3*, alpha-IFN 5.0; *4*, gamma-IFN 8.0; *5*, gamma-IFN 80.0; *6*, alpha-IFN 0.5/gamma-IFN 8.0; *7*, TNF 500; *8*, alpha-IFN 0.5/TNF 500; *9*, alpha-IFN 5.0/TNF 500; *10*, gamme-IFN 8.0/TNF 500; *11*, gamma-IFN 80.0/TNF 500. Concentrations are given in ng/g. The 28s rRNA bands on the blots were used for standardization and correction (data not shown)

Table 1. Relative integrated optical densities (R.I.O.D.) of basal HLA class I expression of eight different RCC xenografts as measured on autoradiograms. For integration of the basal expression levels, the expression level of the NU-3 tumor (lowest basal class I expression) was given the value 1

Tumor	NC-65	NU-1	NU-3	NU-5	NU-10	NU-12	NU-20	NU-22
R.I.O.D.	1.7	2.5	1.0	38.0	6.0	5.0	1.2	36.0

higher in all groups treated with a combination of two cytokines than in the corresponding single cytokine treated groups.

The NU-5 and NU-22 tumors show a remarkable high class I expression in the untreated control groups (Table 1). The induction of expression upon treatment, however, is relatively low; 3.6 and 2.9 times the control level for both lines respectively upon treatment with alpha-IFN 5.0/TNF 500 ng/g. Upregulation is higher in the IFN/TNF treated groups than in the IFN treated groups and a rise in HLA class I expression is dose dependent for IFN.

The other xenografts tested, NC-65, NU-1, NU-10 and NU-12, have an intermediate basal expression of HLA class I. Inducibility of HLA class I expression in NC-65 and NU-1 was absent or moderate in the single cytokine treated groups. All combinations of the IFNs with TNF, however, result in a rise in class I expression and, again, maximum modulation of expression in these tumours is measured in the alpha-IFN 5.0/TNF 500 ng/g treated groups.

Differences in HLA class I expression on the NU-10 and NU-12 tumour lines (Fig. 1a) are pronounced. Highest modulation of class I expression is again shown by the alpha-IFN 5.0/TNF 500 ng/g treated groups, which show a 10 to 12-fold rise in the expression. Most combination groups show higher class I expression than the single cytokine treated groups. Also in these tumours, upregulation of class I is highest in the groups treated with the highest IFN dose.

HLA Class II Expression in Untreated and Cytokine Treated Renal Tumor Xenografts

Five of the eight lines, i.e. the NC-65, NU-1, NU-3, NU-5, and NU-20 lines, show no visible HLA class II expression, neither in the untreated controls nor in any of the cytokine treated groups (Fig. 2). Interestingly, in the NU-1 tumor, class II expression appeared to be inducible to detectable levels by gamma-IFN.

The NU-10 tumor shows a class II expression in the control group which can be strongly modulated by alpha- and gamma-IFN (Figs. 1, 2). TNF cannot modulate HLA class II expression on this tumor; however, for alpha-IFN the combinations with TNF show a more pronounced augmentation than the alpha-IFN treated groups. Augmentation of class II expression is dose dependent in the range tested and most pronounced for the gamma-IFN treated groups (Fig. 2).

Treatment of the NU-12 tumor results in upregulation of class II expression by all treatment modalities except for TNF and only a minor rise in expression is noticed with the low alpha-IFN dose. Again, upregulation is dependent on the IFN dosage. Also in this tumor line, TNF has dual effects on class II expression. TNF itself has no effect on class II expression, whereas relative class II expression in the alpha-IFN treated groups is upregulated by TNF. As for the NU-10 and NU-12 tumor lines, stimulation of class II expression on the NU-22 tumor is noticed for alpha- as well as for gamma-IFN and, again, TNF has no effect on HLA class II expression on this line when tested as single cytokine. However, although differences are small, it further enhances upregulation of class II by alpha-IFN. Also for this tumor, strongest modulation of class II expression is found in the groups treated with highest IFN doses.

Relation Between the Expression and Inducibility of HLA Antigens and Sensitivity to Cytokine Therapy

Having found that HLA class I and class II antigens can be differentially modulated in vivo we evaluated whether basal expression levels and/or inducibility *in general* were related to cytokine sensitivity. Relative basal expression levels were quantified by northern analyses (Table 1). Upon comparison with the sensitivity of the tumor lines for cytokine treatment (Beniers et al. 1991), it is evident that there is poor correlation between basal class I expression and the sensitivity for cytokine treatment. Similarly, for class II expression, as far as present on the untreated tumors, the correlation between basal expression and sensitivity was poor, too.

We compared inducibility in general of both class I and class II HLA antigens with the sensitivity for the cytokines. It appears that, at least for the direct effects of the cytokines, there is a direct relation between sensitivity of the lines and the level of upregulation of both classes of antigens. Both sensitive tumors NU-10 and NU-12 show high upregulation of both class I and class II antigens, whereas the insensitive tumours NU-3 and NU-20 show only low upregulation of both class I and class II antigens. All other lines which show intermediate sensitivity for the cytokines also show intermediate upregulation of class I and class II antigens. Also, the NU-22 tumour shows low upregulation of class I antigens but high upregulation of the class II antigens. Nevertheless, this tumor seems to be only moderately sensitive for the direct effects of the cytokines. So, substantial upregulation of both class I and class II antigen is apparently indicative for a good response to cytokine treatment. Upregulation of either class I or class II correlates with a moderate sensitivity of that tumor line.

Short-term In Vitro Culture Test

We first tested cells of the xenografts, and results of the in vitro and in vivo treatments closely resembled each other in terms of HLA class I and II expression. Some primary renal tumours have been tested by this method; however, the predictive value for response can only be evaluated after full treatment of the patients.

Discussion

In this study we evaluated the usefulness of HLA class I and class II expression on RCC xenografts as predictive markers for response to cytokine therapy. Since expression of HLA class I and class II antigens is directly related to the functionality of CD8+ and CD4+ T lymphocytes, which play an important role in the defense mechanism of the body against alloand abnormal autoantigens, optimal modulation of the class I and class II antigens may be important in host reactivity against cancer cells. However, in the T cell deficient nude mouse, T cell mediated effector mechanisms cannot be studied. Hence, *no functional relation* between class I and class II modulation and cytokine induced antitumor effects can be established.

Figure 2 shows that all xenografts show upregulation of HLA class I expression after treatment with alpha-IFN, gamma-IFN, TNF and/ or combinations of them. It also shows that considerable differences in the extent of modulation exist between the different tumors. In general, a dose-response relationship between upregulation of the HLA class I antigens and IFN concentration (in the dose range tested) was evident. Comparing these results with the in vivo sensitivity of the tumors for the different cytokine treatments [4], in which it was found that some of the tumors showed stronger growth inhibition when treated with the low IFN dose than with the high IFN dose, it becomes clear that in this model the maximum rise in HLA class I expression is not related to highest sensitivity of the xenografts for a particular treatment regimen.

As far as HLA class II expression is detectable in the untreated control groups, and within the dose range tested, HLA class II upregulation is also related to the alpha- and gamma-IFN concentration in a typical dose-response relationship.

When we focus on the individual cytokines, it becomes clear that alpha-IFN has the strongest effect on class I HLA antigen expression. Gamma-IFN and TNF also induce the expression of these molecules, albeit to a lesser extent. Noticeably, maximum induction of class I expression is always found for the combination of alpha-IFN 5.0/TNF 500, irrespective of the effect on tumor growth. Class II expression is influenced predominantly by gamma-IFN. Alpha-IFN also has a clear effect on expression of these molecules, whereas TNF has no such effect at all. In combinations of TNF with the interferons, however, a differential effect was observed. Whereas TNF did not add to the effect when combined with gamma-IFN, it resulted in a stronger relative induction of class II expression when combined with alpha-IFN. Again, for the inducibility of class II expression, the highest achievable effect on tumor growth did not correlate with the maximum rise in expression of class II expression at a given treatment regimen. So, apparently the inducibility at a given dosage was not indicative for the corresponding response to therapy. When we scored for inducibility in general, however, it became evident that this correlated well with cytokine therapy for a given tumor line.

We, therefore, conclude that the basal expression levels of class I and class II antigens does not predict effects of these cytokines on growth of that particular line. In a clinical setting, it was also found that there is no significant correlation between pretreatment HLA-DR expression status of a tumor and subsequent response to therapy. Irrespective of the basal expression level, however, our studies showed that the extent of augmentation of both HLA class I and class II antigens were indicative for the response of renal tumor xenografts towards alpha-IFN, gamma-IFN and TNF. We showed here that in a model in which no T cell mediated effector mechanisms are active, there is a good correlation between both HLA class I and class II antigen expression and the sensitivity of a particular tumor for the direct cytostatic effects of alpha-IFN, gamma-IFN and TNF. Because T cell effector mechanisms cannot explain these results, modulation of the HLA class I and class II antigens here probably function as predictive markers for response as "innocent bystander," indicating that mechanisms of a cytokine mediated induction of expression can be activated. Concomitantly with induction of the HLA class I and II antigens, other antigens not yet studied may be upregulated during therapy, augmenting and or inducing for instance monocyte/ macrophage responses.

The close resemblance of the in vivo and in vitro HLA class I and II modulation of the tumor lines upon treatment with the cytokines indicates the potential usefulness of the short-term in vitro test. The predictive value of the modulations found on primary tumor cells, however, can only be evaluated after full treatment of the patients, but this test eventually might predict response of the patients towards cytokine therapy and may be useful in selecting patients for clinical trials.

References

1. Auffray C, Rougeon W (1980) Purification of mouse immunoglobulin heavy-chain messenger RNAs from total myeloma tumor RNA. Eur J Biochem 107: 303–314
2. Aulitzky W, Gastl G, Aulitzky WE, et al. (1990) Successful treatment of metastatic renal cell carcinoma with a biologically active dose of recombinant interferon-gamma. J Clin Oncol 7: 1875–1884
3. Barnstable CJ, Bodmer WF, Brown G, Galfre G, Milstein C, Williams AF, Ziegler A (1978) Production of monoclonal antibodies to group A erythrocytes, HLA and other human cell surface antigens- New tools for genetic analysis. Cell 14: 9–20
4. Beniers AJMC, van Moorselaar RJA, Peelen WP, Debruyne FMJ, Schalken JA (1991) Differential sensitivity of renal cell carcinoma xenografts towards therapy with interferon-alpha, interferon-gamma, tumor necrosis factor and their combinations. Urol Res 19: 91–98
5. Beniers AJMC, Peelen WP, Schaafsma HE, Beck JLM, Debruyne FMJ, Schalken JA (1991) Establishment and characterization of five new renal tumor xenografts. Am J Path (in press)
6. Höehn W, Schroeder FH (1978) Renal cell carcinoma: two new cell lines and a serially transplantable nude mouse tumor (NC-65). Invest Urol 16: 106–112
7. Lemonnier FA, Rebai N, le Bouteiller PP, Malissen B, Caillol DH, Kourilsky FM (1982) Epitopic analysis of detergent-solubilized HLA molecules by solid-phase radioimmunoassay. J Immunol Methods 54: 9–22
8. Rubin JT, Elwood LJ, Rosenberg SA, Lotze MT (1989) Immunohistochemical correlates of response to recombinant interleukin-2-based immunotherapy in humans. Cancer Res 49: 7086–7092

9. Seakaly RP, Tonnelle C, Strubin M, Mach B, Long EO (1986) Cell surface expression of class II histocompatibility antigens occur in the absence of the invariant chain. J Exp Med 164: 1490–1504
10. Sood AK, Pereira D, Weissman SM (1981) Isolation and partial nucleotide sequence of a cDNA clone for human histocompatibility antigen HLA-B by use of an oligodeoxynucleotide primer. Proc Natl Acad Sci USA 78: 616–620

Alien Gene Transfection and the Immune Response to Tumors*

P. Frost[1]

The treatment of metastatic cancer remains the preeminent problem in neoplasia. Despite significant advances in our understanding of some of the molecular mechanisms in carcinogenesis and tumor progression, our ability to translate these findings into clinical treatment remains limited. While these molecular studies evolve, the more immediate need for new treatment modalities has led to a more intense evaluation of current approaches to therapy, including surgery, radiation and chemotherapy. In addition, we have also seen a resurgent interest in immunotherapy, which has led to promising approaches in some diseases. Unfortunately, the goal of developing specific systemic immunotherapy remains elusive. In this manuscript we will describe some ideas we have used in our attempt to treat established metastases in murine models.

The Nature of Tumor Antigens

It is generally accepted that tumor antigens exist. This is particularly true for murine tumors where evidence for such antigens derives from multiple studies. One of the best examples of tumor antigen expression are the experiments of Boon et al. and Frost et al. [1, 2, 8, 9]. In these cumulative studies, eight different murine tumors were treated with mutagens (EMS or MNNG) or hypomethylating agents (5-Aza-C and 5-Aza-CdR) cloned and selected for their inability to grow in syngeneic hosts. These Imm^+ clones were not tumorigenic in

* Supported in part by PHS Grants 38853 and 41525 and The Sid Richardson Foundation

[1] The University of Texas M.D. Anderson Cancer Center, Department of Cell Biology, Houston, TX 77030, USA

G. Staehler S. Pomer (Eds.)
Basic and Clinical Research on Renal Cell Carcinoma

normal hosts at challenge doses two to three times greater than the dose of parent tumor cells required to induce tumor growth. The clones did grow in nude mice [8, 9]. Imm^+ clones were able to engender a specific cytotoxic T lymphocytes (CTL) response further supporting the immunologic basis for their lack of tumorigenicity in normal animals.

While these studies raise a number of questions, I will address only two. The first relates to the long held view that tumors are heterogeneous [4, 10] and it is therefore illogical to attempt to engender an immune response capable of dealing with all the potential antigens in any tumor cell population. The mutagen-induced Imm^+ variant studies prove that this view is overly pessimistic. In all those studies unique Imm^+ clones were able to induce protective responses against the parent tumor, meaning that all the cells within the parent tumor share a common antigen though they are likely heterogeneous for numerous other phenotypes. This observation encourages a more optimistic view regarding specific immunotherapy.

A second issue raised by these experiments relates to the question of the nature of tumor antigens. Since the cells of the murine tumors tested all expressed an antigen unique for that tumor (as shown by the rejection of all parent tumor cells after immunization with a single Imm^+ clone), why were these antigens incapable of engendering a response to themselves? We propose that this failure of tumor antigens to engender an immune response is due to their "hapten-like" nature. In classic immunologic studies haptens are defined as being antigenic but not immunogenic. Thus, if a hapten is linked to a carrier molecule, it will induce a response while it cannot do so on its own. Furthermore, once antibody to the hapten is produced, it will interact with the hapten. While hapten-carrier models are generally defined serologically (humoral immunity) rather than by cellular immune responses, they do provide a reasonable analogy for what is observed with tumor antigens.

The analogy is further supported by concept of associative recognition as first presented by Lake and Mitchison [14] and experimentally defined by Keene and Foreman [13]. These latter authors showed that congenic strains of mice differing in the expression of a single allele could not engender a rejection response against each other's tissues. However, if male mouse tissue bearing the H-Y antigen in addition to the single allelic difference were used in immunization, a strong rejection response was induced. The concept of associative recognition supports the view that at least two antigenic signals are needed to induce a response to cell surface antigens.

The experiments with mutagen-induced Imm^+ variants implied that mutagen treatment likely leads to the expression of a "new" antigen that serves as the second surface antigen needed to induce a response to the parent tumor antigen. This hypothesis has recently been proven by Sibille et al. [16], who showed these to be altered (due to a point mutation) normal proteins.

These studies provided a basis for our experiments, in which the aim was to provide a second surface antigen or other modifying factor without the need for mutagen treatment.

Alien Gene Transfection

Studies with the Hemagglutinin Antigen of Influenza Virus

Hemagglutinin antigen (HA) studies are reviewed in detail elsewhere in this book (Schackert and Frost). Let it suffice to say that the expression of HA on the surface of a number of murine tumors (CT-26 colon adenocarcinoma [6], SPI spontaneous mammary carcinoma and the RBL-5 rhabdomyosarcoma) resulted in the generation of immunogenic variants that could protect against a challenge with parental tumor cells. This system offered the advantage of providing the ability to select high HA expressers using a fluorescence-activated cell sorter (FACS). In addition, HA-expressing cells retained their immunogenicity after X-irradiation [11]. These latter two issues are of some importance for the potential transfer of this technology to the clinic.

Transfection with the Interleukin-2 Gene

We reasoned that if a second antigen such as HA can enhance the response to murine tumor antigens by possibly providing T-cell help, then providing a lymphokine such as interleukin 2 (IL-2) could achieve the same goal [7]. CT-26 colon tumor cells were transfected with the pBCMG-neo-IL-2 plasmid that contains a cytomegalovirus (CMV) promoter the neo and murine IL-2 genes. The transfected cells were then selected in geneticin and subsequently assessed for IL-2 production using the assay originally described by Janis et al. [12] CT-26/IL-2 cells were then injected s.c. into Balb/c mice at doses ranging from 1×10^4 to 1×10^7 cells/mouse. While parent CT-26 cells will grow in 100% of animals at a challenge dose of 1×10^3 cells, no growth occurred at doses of CT-26/IL-2 when 1×10^4 or 1×10^5 cells were injected. At 1×10^6, only 2 of 55 animals had tumors and even at a challenge dose of 1×10^7, only 4 of 15 animals developed tumors. This dramatic increase in immunogenicity was also able to produce protection against a challenge with nontransfected parental cells. In an effort to understand the mechanism of the CT-26/IL-2 induced immune response, we proceeded to demonstrate that CT-26/IL-2 can engender a CTL response that can be abrogated by treatment of the effector cells with anti CD4 but not anti-CD8 antibodies. In addition, CT-26/IL-2 cells were able to grow in animals that were treated in vivo with anti-CD8 antibodies. Animals treated with anti-CD4 remained capable of rejecting a CT-26/IL-2 challenge [7].

Similar results were obtained with two additional tumors. However, while the B16/IL-2 [7] and SP1/IL-2 (Frost, unpublished) tumors failed to grow in syngeneic animals, they could not protect against a challenge with parental cells. This could relate to the fact that both of these tumors express five-to tenfold less class I MHC antigen than the CT-26 tumor. The issue of the role of class I in the rejection of parental tumors is presented in detail elsewhere and will be discussed in part, in relation to interferon (IFN)-γ production by SP1 cells.

These findings support the view that the local (paracrine) production of IL-2 by tumor cells bypasses the requirement for T-helper cells and allows for the direct activation of effector (cytotoxic) T cells. The presence of IL-2 in the local environment overcomes the need for the production of some cytokines by T-helper cells and allows hapten-like tumor antigens to be recognized. In short, the paracrine production of IL-2 appears to fulfill the functions of the carrier antigen and is believed to enhance T-helper cell function.

Transfection with IFN-γ

The question of the role of class I major histocompatibility complex (MHC) in tumor immunogenicity remains incompletely resolved [3, 17]. While some have argued that class I MHC antigens are essential for an immune response to murine tumors, it is also well known that many murine tumors express high levels of class I MHC but remain tumorigenic (witness the CT-26 tumor).

It is also well established that many murine tumors that do not express MHC antigens can be induced to do so by treatment with IFN-γ. The effects of IFN-γ on MHC expression persists for as long as it remains in the media. Removal of IFN-γ results in a loss of MHC expression within 24–48 h. With this in mind, we designed a series of studies to determine whether the continuous production of IFN-γ by non-class I-expressing tumor cells would enhance their tumorigenicity.

SP1 tumor cells were cotransfected with the murine IFN-γ gene using a CMV expression vector (provided by Dr. T. Sakata) and pSV2-neo. After selection in geneticin, eight individual culture plates were screened for IFN-γ production using the method described by Mory et al. [15]. The three lines found to produce IFN-γ, 1C, 3C and 6L, secreted 16, 32 and 256 U/ml, respectively. When injected into syngeneic animals 1C and 3C grew in a manner identical to parent SP1 cells [5]. However, 6L cells failed to grow at challenge doses exceeding 1×10^6 cells. (Parent SP1 cells consistantly produce tumors at challenge doses of 1×10^3.)

6L cells also engendered a cytotoxic response, but this was non-specific, for only nylon wool adherent cells were cytotoxic. Nylon wool nonadherent cells produced a much lower cytotoxic response. In addition, the CTL in the spleens of 6L immunized mice were not depleted by treatment with anti-CD4, anti-CD8 or anti-CD3 antibodies.

6L cells did grow in nude mice producing tumors which when recultured in vitro produced varying amounts of IFN-γ. Two of these tumors were assessed for class I MHC (6LA: 256 U/ml; 6LB-8 U/ml) and both expressed equivalent levels of MHC as measured by FACS. This finding argued that it is the expression of high levels of IFN-γ rather than class I MHC expression that is responsible for the failure of SP1/IFN-γ cells to grow in vivo. This was further substantiated by the fact that CT-26 cells that constitutively express class I MHC antigens and grow progressively; failed to grow when secreting IFN-γ.

Despite their ability to engender an immune response CBA/IFN-γ could only protect against a weak challenge with parental SP1 cells (1×10^4). It is likely that factors unrelated to class I expression or IFN-γ production alone or in combination are sufficient to induce a protective response against a parent tumor challenge.

Discussion and Future Directions

The treatment of neoplasia by activation of a systemic immune response remains an estimable goal. Unfortunately, our success to date has been both disappointing and frustrating. Approaches which targeted tumors using non-specific, broad immune stimulation with

Bacillus Calmette-Guérin (BCG) or, more recently, systemic administration of massive doses of lymphokines have not resulted in any major changes in response rates in most solid tumors. However, some effects, particularly in some leukemias, are worth making note of.

The approaches reviewed in this article offer an alternative design for stimulating an immune response to tumors. They are based on certain fundemental ideas that include the views that:

1. Tumors express unique antigens.
2. Tumor antigens have a limited repertoire, i.e., tumor heterogeneity may not be a limitation to the development of immunotherapy.
3. Tumor antigens are "hapten-like" and require assistance in generating a T-cell helper response.
4. This can be achieved via "associative recognition" by the expression of a second antigen on the cell surface or by bypassing the need for T-cell help by providing a means for the tumor to secrete lymphokines in a "paracrine" fashion.

While these early studies are promising, difficulties have yet to be overcome. The failure of SP1/IL-2, B16/IL-2 and SP1/IFN-γ to induce protective responses against the parent tumor implies that other more effective antigens, lymphokines or combinations of both will have to be developed. The adaptation of these methods to human disease will have to overcome the problem of customizing cells for individual patients. This will require an ability to establish cell lines from each patient, a formidable task. In addition, it will be necessary to only use immunizing cells that are incapable of replication. While this is readily overcome by irradiating HA-expressing cells, in our hands IL-2 or IFN-γ producing cells generally lose their effectiveness as immunogens when X-irradiated.

These difficulties, while complicating, should not be insurmountable. A number of modifications of published methods are already at hand and novel approaches using retroviral vectors have proven themselves very effective.

We have recently used combinations of murine tumor cells expressing HA and secreting IL-2 or IFN-γ in the hope of engendering more rapid responses to murine tumors. We have seen considerable improvement in the treatment of metastases but the results are not yet optimal. This is likely because murine tumor models are excessively aggressive. It is important to recall that murine tumors may indeed grow rapidly in direct proportion to the life span of a mouse (2 years); but the initiation of their immune response takes about as long as it does in humans, where nonleukemic tumor growth is generally not as explosive. Thus the difficulty in treating established metastases in mice may not truly reflect on the usefulness of these approaches in human neoplasia.

It would appear that the revolution in molecular genetic technology may be beginning to influence the diagnosis and treatment of human disease. Alien gene transfection or infection with retroviral vectors could herald the advent of new approaches to immunotherapy.

References

1. Boon T, Kellerman O (1977) Rejection by syngeneic mice of cell variants obtained by mutagenesis of a malignant teratocarcinoma cell line. Proc Natl Acad Sci 74: 272–275
2. Boon T (1983) Antigenic tumor cell variants obtained with mutagens. Adv Cancer Res 39: 121–151
3. Carlow DA, Kerbel RS, Elliott BE (1989) Failure of expression of class I major histocompatibility antigens to alter tumor immunogenicity of a spontaneous murine carcinoma. J Natl Cancer Inst 81: 759–767
4. Dexter DL, Calabresi P (1982) Intraneoplastic diversity. Biochem Biophys Acta 695: 97–112
5. Esumi N, Hunt B, Itaya T, Frost P (1991) The reduced tumorigenicity of murine tumor cells secreting interferon gamma is due to non-specific host responses and is unrelated to class I MHC expression. Cancer Res 51: 1185–1189
6. Fearon ER, Itaya T, Hunt B, Vogelstein B, Frost P (1988) Induction in a murine tumor of immunogenic tumor variants by transfection with a foreign gene. Cancer Res 48: 2975–2980
7. Fearon ER, Pardoll DM, Itaya T, et al. (1990) Interleukin-2 production by tumor cells bypasses T helper function in the generation of an antitumor response. Cell 60: 397–403
8. Frost P, Kerbel R, Bauer E, Tartamella-Biondo R, Cefalu W (1978) Mutagen treatment as a means for selecting immunogenic variants from otherwise poorly immunogenic malignant tumors. Cancer Res 43: 125–132
9. Frost P, Liteplo RG, Donaghue TP, Kerbel RS (1984) Selection of strongly immunogenic "Tum" variants from tumors at high frequency using 5-azacytidine. J Exp Med 159: 1491–1501
10. Heppner GH (1984) Tumor heterogeneity. Cancer Res 44: 2259–2265
11. Itaya T, Hunt B, Frost P (1989) Retention of immunogenicity after X-irradiation of mouse colon tumor cells expression the transfected influenze virus hemagglutinin gene. Cancer Immunol Immunother 28: 248–252
12. Janis E, Kaufmann SE, Schwartz RH, Pardoll DM (1989) Activation of gamma/delta T cells in the primary immune response to *Mycobacterium tuberculosis*. Science 244: 713–716
13. Kerve JA, Foreman J (1982) Helper activity is required for the in vivo generation of cytotoxic T lymphocytes. J Exp Med 155: 768–782

14. Lake P, Mitchinson NA (1976) Associative control of the immune response to cell surface antigens. Immunol Commun 5: 795–805
15. Mory Y, Chernajovsky Y, Feinstein SI, et al. (1981) Synthesis of human interferon β_1 in *Escherichia coli* infected by a lambda phage recombinant containing a human genomic fragment. Eur J Biochem 120: 197–202
16. Sibille C, Chomez P, Wildmann C, et al. (1990) Structure of the gene of tum transplantation antigen P198: a point mutation generates a new antigenic peptide. J Exp Med 172: 35–45
17. Tanaka E, Isselbacher KS, Khoury G, Jay G (1985) Reversal of oncogenesis by the expression of a major histocompatibility complex class I gene. Science 228: 26–30

Active Specific Immunotherapy with Tumor Cells Expressing a Foreign Gene*

H.K. Schackert[1] and P. Frost[2]

Introduction

Primary malignant tumors can be surgically resected; this results either in a definitive eradication of the neoplasm or in a local or metastatic recurrence. Surgery remains the principal treatment with a curative intent. Although surgical techniques have been refined in recent years there is no clear evidence that this might have a beneficial impact on survival rates [6]. Local or regional recurrence of colorectal cancer, for example, may be due to tumor cells disseminating from the primary tumor via the draining lymphatics. Thus liver metastases result from small tumor aggregates that likely exist but are not detectable at the time of surgery.

Since the efficiency of surgery is limited by the ability of tumors to metastasize, there is a need for adjuvant treatment modalities that are capable of reaching all sites of possible metastatic spread. With few exceptions radiotherapy and chemotherapy have not improved survival rates. New experimental approaches, possibly including molecular biology techniques, could be effective in designing novel immunotherapeutic modes of treatment.

The aim of this study was to develop experimental tumor models that closely mimic the clinical situation of colon cancer metastasis. Based on these animal models a recently described approach for increasing the immunogenicity of tumor cells [1] was used to protect

* Supported by the scholarships Scha 413/1-1 and Scha 413/1-2 from the Deutsche Forschungsgemeinschaft, Bonn, Germany

[1] Chirurgische Universitätsklinik, Abteilung 2.1.1., Im Neuenheimer Feld 110, W-6900 Heidelberg, FRG
[2] The University of Texas M.D. Anderson Cancer Center, Department of Cell Biology, Houston, TX 77030, USA

G. Staehler S. Pomer (Eds.)
Basic and Clinical Research on Renal Cell Carcinoma

against the development or treat established metastases of a murine colon adenocarcinoma (CT-26) with syngeneic tumor cells expressing the transfected hemagglutinin antigen (HA) of human influenza virus. It has been shown that tumor cells expressing HA not only fail to grow in syngeneic hosts but also elicit an immune response that is cross protective against a s.c. challenge with non-transfected parent CT-26 cells [1].

The underlying mechanism of increased immunogenicity of the tumor associated antigen (TAA) in the presence of HA has been explained by the concept of associate recognition defined by Lake and Mitchison [9] and Keene and Forman [7]. The nature of the TAA may be "hapten-like" and therefore antigenic but not immunogenic [2]. By introducing an additional immunogenic "carrier-like" viral antigen on the surface of the tumor cell an immunological response is engendered against both the viral and TAA.

In this report we show that immunization with CT-26 cells expressing high levels of HA (clone 5) protects against CT-26 tumor challenge in the cecum, the lymph system of the cecum, the liver and the lung, but not in the brain. The response to s.c. immunization is specific, long lasting and can be transferred by immune cells of preimmunized animals. Furthermore active specific immunotherapy of established micrometastases can be achieved in the lung but not in the liver of syngeneic mice.

Material and Methods

CT-26 cells were co-transfected with the plasmid vectors pSV2neo and pBV-1MTHA (a bovine papilloma virus expression vector containing the murine metallothionein promoter, MT, and the HA gene of the A/Jap/305/57 H2N2 strain of human influenza virus). After selection in geneticin, HA-antigen expressing cells were sorted three times using a fluorescence-activated cell sorter (FACS). These cells (FACS-3) were cloned by limiting dilution and single colonies were harvested and propagated as clones. Clone 5 and clone 18 were high expressors of HA and were shown to induce a cross protective immune response against nontransfected parent CT-26 cells injected s.c. [1].

As few as 10^3 CT-26 cells injected s.c. results in progressive tumor growth in 50% of the animals [1], supporting the view that CT-26 tumor cells are poorly to moderately immunogenic [1]. Recent experiments have shown that the immunogenicity of the TAA of CT-26 cells correlates with the expression of HA on the surface of the tumor cell. CT-26 cells which are low expressors of HA are tumorigenic while high expressors of HA are immunogenic; 1×10^7 HA-expressing CT-26 cells injected s.c. fail to grow in syngeneic hosts [1]. The tumorigenicity of these cells, which had been selected by repeated FACS, is over 10000 times lower than that of the nontransfected parent CT-26 tumor cells. The immunogenicity of high HA expressor clone 5 cells used in these experiments was 13-fold greater than parental cells [5]. Additionally, X-irradiation does not impair the immunogenicity of HA expressing cells [4].

Metastases were selectively induced in the cecum and the lymph system of the cecum, the liver, the lung and the brain by injecting tumor cell suspensions into the lymphoid follicle of the cecum [11], the portal vein, the tail vein and the internal carotid artery [10], respectively. In all protection experiments animals were immunized twice by injecting viable clone 5 cells s.c. at doses of 1×10^6 and 1×10^5 3 weeks and 1 week before challenge with parent CT-26 cells as micrometastases in various organs. In all experiments aimed at treating established metastases, animals were first challenged with CT-26 cells in the liver or lung. Three days later (when micrometastases were found by histological examination) immunization was begun with 5×10^6 irradiated (12000 rad) clone 5 cells given s.c. followed by a second s.c. injection of the same cells 7 days later.

Results

Protection against metastases in the cecum, lymph system of the cecum, liver and lung was successful in all experiments carried out using the above immunization schedule. While 5×10^4 CT-26 cells injected into the cecum produced tumors in 8 of 10 animals after 32 days, all 10 animals immunized before challenge were free of tumor. The same number of CT-26 cells injected into the portal vein produced a median number and range of 131 (17–over 150) metastases in 12 of 12 animals after 21 days. In contrast the median and range in the preimmunized animals was 0 (0–104) and the tumor incidence 25%. Similar results were obtained protecting against lung metastases [12].

Further experiments showed that preimmunization with clone 5 was not effective against the production of CT-26 brain metastases. Nine of nine animals developed brain tumors and died within 14–19 days after challenge with 1×10^5 CT-26 cells into the internal carotid artery, and all eight preimmunized animals died after 17–19 days of brain tumor. Autopsy and histological examination revealed that all control animals or preimmunized animals had similar tumor growth in the choroid plexus of the ventricle and in the parenchyma of the brain without lymphocytic infiltrates.

Additional experiments confirmed that the protective response of clone 5 immunization meets the criteria for an immune response. It is specific, establishes a specific memory response and can be transferred by spleen lymphocytes of animals immunized repeatedly with clone 5 cells. Histological examination of rejection of s.c. injected parent CT-26 cells in preimmunized animals showed a massive influx of mononuclear cells followed by tumor necrosis and replacement by fibrosis within 11 days.

Active specific immunotherapy (ASI) and consequent eradication of established metastases is a far more challenging task than protection against tumor challenge in different organs. The ASI experiments focused on liver and lung, which are most often the targets of metastatic spread in colorectal cancer. Two different experiments had shown that ASI with irradiated parent CT-26 as a vaccine has no effect on the growth of established CT-26 lung metastases and survival of the animals compared to nontreated control animals. Therefore in all the following experiments nontreated mice were used as controls instead of CT-26 treated animals. Several experiments confirmed that ASI with clone 5 in the above mentioned schedule could eradicate established metastases in the lung. Success depended on the tumor burden at the time of the first immunization and on the immunization dose. Experiments starting immunization on day 6 instead of day 3 were much less effective. For example 10 of 10 nontreated control animals challenged with 20000 CT-26 tumor cells via the tail vein developed lung metastases within 60 days. In addition all animals immunized with clone 5 beginning on day 6 after challenge developed lung metastases, whereas 5 of 10 animals which had the first immunization on day 3 after CT-26 challenge were free of tumor at that time.

All experiments with the same immunization schedule used to treat liver metastases failed. There was no benefit in survival from ASI with clone 5 in animals bearing established liver metastases. In contrast to the production of lung metastases the establishment of liver metastases requires anesthesia and laparotomy to inject the cells into the portal vein. These procedures have been shown to impair the immune system and might represent an explanation for our failure to successfully treat liver metastases.

Discussion and Conclusion

Increased immunogenicity of TAA can be achieved by xenogenization of the tumor cell with foreign antigens introduced by infecting the cell with a virus [8, 13] or by transfection with a viral gene whose product is expressed on the cell surface [1]. This effect has been explained by an increased production of T helper cells [3] as a result of "associative recognition" [7, 9]. The response engendered by the alien gene is not only directed against the foreign antigen but also against the TAA.

Transfection of CT-26 tumor cells with the hemagglutinin gene of influenza virus and high expression of the gene product on the cell surface increased the immunogenicity of the CT-26 tumor cells 13-fold [5]. High expressor cells, like clone 5, were not only potent immunogens for the protection against a CT-26 challenge in different organs, but were also useful in treating established metastases in the lung. The advantage of conserving immunogenicity of transfected cells after irradiation with 12 000 rad is a prerequisite for the potential use of such system in the clinical arena. Several possibilities exist to improve ASI with xenogenized tumor cells. More effective antigens alone or in combination have to be tested. Furthermore the production and secretion of lymphokines as tools to increase immunogenicity of tumor cells are reviewed in this book (Frost). In summary, local and systemic production of antigens and cytokines achieved by transfection of benign or tumor cells may not only provide insights into the mechanisms of immune defense of neoplasms but also give rise to new strategies in fighting cancer with immunotherapeutic approaches.

References

1. Fearon ER, Itaya T, Hunt B, Vogelstein B, Frost P (1988) Induction in a murine tumor of immunogenic tumor variants by transfection with a foreign gene. Cancer Res 38: 2975–2980
2. Frost P, Chernojovsky Y (1990) Transformation injury and the unicellular phenotype of malignant cells. Cancer Metast Rev 9: 93–97
3. Fujiwara H, Shimizu Y, Takai Y, Wakamiya N, Ueda S, Kato S, Hamaoka T (1984) The augmentation of tumor-specific immunity by virus help. I. Demonstration of vaccinia virus-reactive helper T cell activity involved in enhanced induction of cytotoxic T lymphocyte and antibody responses. Eur J Immunol 14: 171–175
4. Itaya T, Hunt B, Frost P (1989) Retention of immunogenicity after X-irradiation of mouse colon tumor cells expressing the transfected influenza virus hemagglutinin gene. Cancer Immunol Immunother 28: 248–252

5. Itaya T, Schackert HK, Frost P (1989a) The potential immunoregulation of metastases: the use of transfection to produce immunogenic tumor cells. Prog Clin Biol Res 288: 271–279
6. Jeekel J (1987) Can radical surgery improve survival in colorectal cancer? World J Surg 11: 412–417
7. Keene JA, Forman J (1982) Helper activity is required for the in vivo generation of cytotoxic T lymphocytes. J Exp Med 155: 768–782
8. Kobayashi H, Sendo F, Shirai T, Kaji H, Kodama T, Saito H (1969) Modification in growth of transplantable rat tumors exposed to Friend virus. J Natl Cancer Inst 42: 413–419
9. Lake P, Mitchison NA (1976) Associative control of the immune response to cell surface antigens. Immunol Commun 5: 795–805
10. Schackert G, Fidler IJ (1988) Development of in vivo models for studies of brain metastases. Int J Cancer 41: 589–594
11. Schackert HK, Fidler IJ (1989) Development of an animal model to study the biology of recurrent colorectal cancer originating from mesenteric lymph system metastases. Int J Cancer 44: 177–181
12. Schackert HK, Itaya T, Schackert G, Fearon E, Vogelstein B, Frost P (1989) Systemic immunity against a murine colon tumor (CT-26) produced by immunization with syngeneic cells expressing a transfected viral gene product. Int J Cancer 43: 823–827
13. Schirrmacher V, Heicappell R (1987) Prevention of metastatic spread by postoperative immunotherapy with virally modified autologous tumor cells. II. Establishment of specific systemic anti-tumor immunity. Clin Expl Metastasis 5: 147–156

Novel Monoclonal Antibody 138H11 Against Human γ-Glutamyl-Transferase: Classification, Histogenesis and Immunoscintigraphy of Renal Tumors

P. Fischer[1,6], R.P. Baum[2], M. Tauber[1], W. Boeckmann[3], S. Störkel[5], S. Weier[4], and J.E. Scherberich[1]

Summary

Monoclonal antibody (mAb) 138H11 was produced against human gamma-glutamyl transferase as a molecular probe for renal cancer. Immunohistochemical analyses of mAb 138H11 revealed its reaction with the brush border of normal kidney cortex as well as with clear cell and chromophilic renal carcinomas. In contrast, renal oncocytomas, chromophobic carcinomas, and Duct-Bellini carcinomas were negative for this antibody. These results support a new approach for the histogenesis and classification of renal tumors. Immunoscintigraphy of tumor bearing human kidneys, perfused with $^{99}Tc^{m}$-labeled mAb 138H11 after nephrectomy, showed enrichment of 138H11 in three of three clear cell carcinomas that was up to seven fold greater than that in the remaining normal kidney cortex. In contrast, examination of an oncocytoma did not reveal any uptake of labeled mAb 138H11. Our results suggest a possible use of mAb 138H11 for pre-, intra-, and postsurgical diagnosis of primary renal tumors and metastases that may indicate further choices of therapy.

[1] Abteilung für Nephrologie
[2] Nuklearmedizin
[3] Urologie und
[4] Pathologie der Universität, Theodor-Stern-Vai 7, W-6000 Frankfurt a.m. 70, FRG
[5] Institut für Pathologie der Universität, Langenbeckstraße, W-6500 Mainz, FRG
[6] Present address: Research Institute of Seripps Clinic, Department of Immunology (13), 10666 North Torrey Pines Road, La Jolla, CA 92037, USA

G. Staehler S. Pomer (Eds.)
Basic and Clinical Research on Renal Cell Carcinoma

Introduction

Antigenic properties of human epithelial renal tumors can be used for diagnostic and therapeutic purposes and to solve classification problems and histogenetic questions. In this regard, a marker enzyme of the proximal tubule of the human kidney [Scherberich et al. 1978], gamma-glutamyl transferase (GGT), also is expressed in renal cell carcinomas (RCC). This enzyme has been proposed as a tumor cell marker [Vanderlaan et al. 1981], and increased or novel forms of GGT have been described for several tumors including RCC [Toya et al. 1983, Hada et al. 1978, Fischer et al. 1990]. To investigate GGT as a possible tumor marker for renal cell carcinoma, we have produced mAbs against human kidney GGT and investigated them as possible tools for the comparative diagnosis of renal cancer.

Materials and Methods

Preparation of mAbs Directed Against GGT

As described earlier [Fischer et al. 1990], spleen cells of Balb/c mice which had been immunized with purified human kidney GGT were fused with X63Ag8.653 myeloma cells by standard hybridoma technology. Hybridomas were hypoxanthine-aminopterin-thymidine (HAT)-selected and screened with a GGT-specific enzyme-linked immunosorbent assay (ELISA) and by immunohistochemistry. The specificity of one of the resulting mAbs, designated 138H11, for human GGT was tested by western blotting and immunoprecipitation assays. The selected hybridoma clone was grown in serum-free medium, supplemented with 3%–10% (v/v) Ultroser HY (growth-factor-containing tissue medium); thus, this mAb could be purified and concentrated in one step by affinity chromatography on protein G-Sepharose.

Immunohistochemistry

Cryosections (<10 µm) of normal human organs and tumors were incubated for 1 h at 25°C with 100 µl of supernatant from the hybridoma producing 138H11 or with control cell culture medium. Bound antibodies were detected with peroxidase-conjugated rabbit-anti-mouse Ig and AEC substrate. Slices were counterstained with hematoxiline. Renal tumors were classified according to Thoenes et al. [1986].

Immunoscintigraphy

MAb 138H11 was labeled with ^{99m}Technecium by the method of Schwarz et al. [1987]. Briefly, purified mAb 138H11 was reduced with mercaptoethanol, lyophilized, and then reacted with a stannous salt component prior to ^{99m}Tc-pertechneate binding. The labeling efficiency was >97%, as determined by instant thin layer chromatography. Tumor-bearing kidneys were perfused with 1 mg ^{99}Tc^{m}-labeled mAb 138H11 (300 MBq) in Euro-Collins solution/20% albumin/methyl-prednisolone for 22 h at under 15°C and then twice for 1 h with the above solution without mAb. The model used was essentially that described by van Dijk et al. [1988]. Perfused kidneys were viewed with a gamma camera (planar and single photo emission computed tomography, SPECT). Tissue sections of interest were measured separately in a gamma-counter and investigated by immunohistochemistry. For details see [Fischer et al. 1991b].

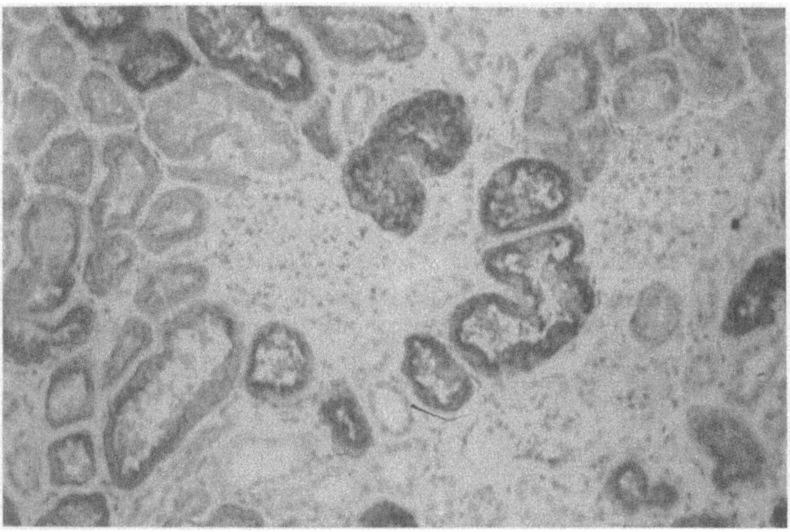

Fig. 1. Normal human kidney. Strong staining with mAb 138H11 of the luminal brush border membrane of the proximal tubule; glomeruli and distal tubules are negative (×100, immunoperoxidase, counterstained with hematoxyline)

Results and Discussion

A number of mAbs to human GGT were produced [Fischer et al. 1989, 1990]. One of these antibodies of IgG1 subclass and designated 138H11, recognizes human kidney GGT by immunohistochemical analyses (Fig. 1) and, in addition, GGT in renal cell carcinomas (Fig. 2). Judging from the binding capacity of mAb 138H11 (Table 1), the different renal tumor types could be clearly divided into two groups: one with nearly 100% positivity including clear cell and chromophilic RCC and another one with 100% negativity (chromophobic RCC, oncocytomas and Duct-Bellini carcinomas).

This binding pattern of mAb 138H11 supports the notion that clear cell and chromophilic RCC, the major portion that makes up all malignant RCC, originates from proximal tubule cells [Störkel and Jacobi 1989]. In parallel, absence of the 138H11 epitope in cell types of the second group confirms that these tumors are not histogenetic derivatives of proximal tubule epithelia [Störkel et al. 1988 and 1989, Ortmann and Vierbuchen 1988, Zerban et al. 1987, Fischer et al. 1991a].

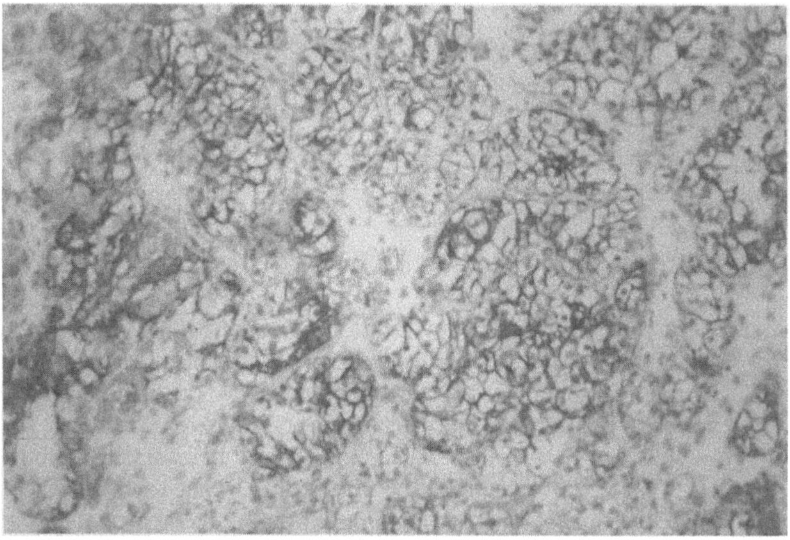

Fig. 2. Renal clear cell carcinoma. Tumor cells strongly express the 138H11 epitope in the contraluminal membrane, whereas stroma cells are negative (×100, hematoxyline)

Table 1. Immunohistochemistry with mAb 138H11 on human organs

Organ	No. pos./tested	Intensity	Remarks
Normal organs:			
Kidney	19/19	+++++	Proximal tubules
Fetal kidney	3/3	++++	Proximal tubules
Colon	0/1	–	–
Colon polyp	1/1	–/+++	Some epithelium
Stomach	1/1	+	Crypts
Liver	3/3	++++	Bile canaliculi
Testicle	1/1	++++	Spermatides
Arteria	0/1	–	–
Muscle	0/1	–	–
Squamous epithelia	0/5	–	–
Thyroid gland	0/1	–	–
Thyroid struma	1/1	+++	Epithelium
Lymphatic ganglion	0/3	–	–
Epithelial renal tumors:			
Clear cell ca.	34/34	+/+++++	Tumor cells
Chromophilic ca.	16/17	+/++++	Tumor cells
Chromophobic ca.	0/9	–	–
Oncocytoma	0/11	–	–
Duct-Bellini ca.	0/1	–	–
Liver metastases	2/2	+/+++	Tumor cells
Other tumors:			
Hepatocell. ca.	1/1	+++++	Tumor cells
Stomach ca.	2/2	++++	Crypts
Squamous cell ca.	0/12	–	–
Pancreas adeno ca.	0/2	–	–

ca., carcinoma

Immunoscintigraphy with MAb 138H11

Immunoscintigraphic tumor localization with mAb 138H11 appeared possible, since in contrast to normal tubule epithelia, kidney tumor cells contain no basement membrane barrier. Three kidneys with clear cell carcinoma and one bearing oncocytoma were perfused with $^{99}Tc^{m}$-labeled mAb 138H11. The kidneys with clear cell carcinomas revealed specific enrichment of the labeled mAb that was up to seven fold greater than that in the remaining normal kidney cortex (Figs. 3, 4). In contrast, the oncocytoma did not show any uptake of the labeled mAb 138H11, and only half of the activity as that found in the kidney cortex was measured in this benign tumor.

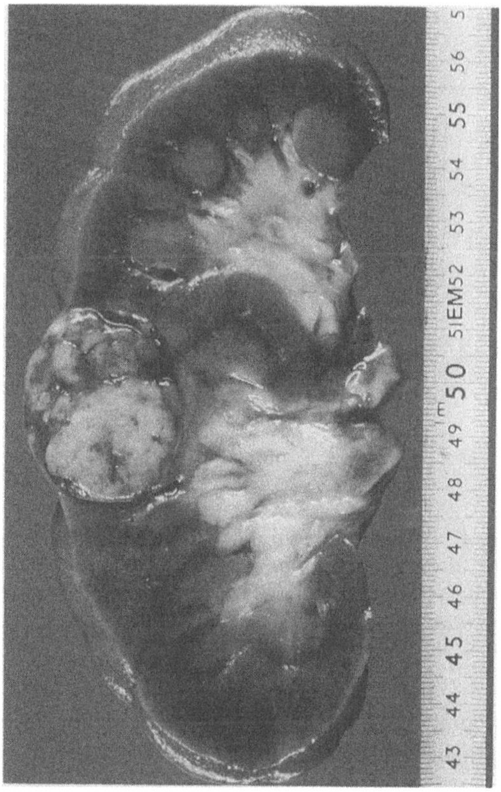

Fig. 3. Macroscopic appearance of a perfused clear cell carcinoma-bearing kidney. The tumor in the cortex region is clearly visible

Immunohistochemical staining of the corresponding tissue sections from these kidneys with peroxidase-labeled anti-mouse Ig serum confirmed the immunoscintigraphic findings. Thus, bound mAb could be demonstrated in the perfused clear cell carcinomas and in the basement membranes of some proximal tubuli in the kidney cortex, whereas the oncocytoma was negative.

Quantitative Immunoassays with MAb 138H11

Different levels of immunoreactive and enzymatically active forms of GGT have been reported for hepatomas [Taniguchi et al. 1985] and were also demonstrated in a pilot study with a competitive ELISA

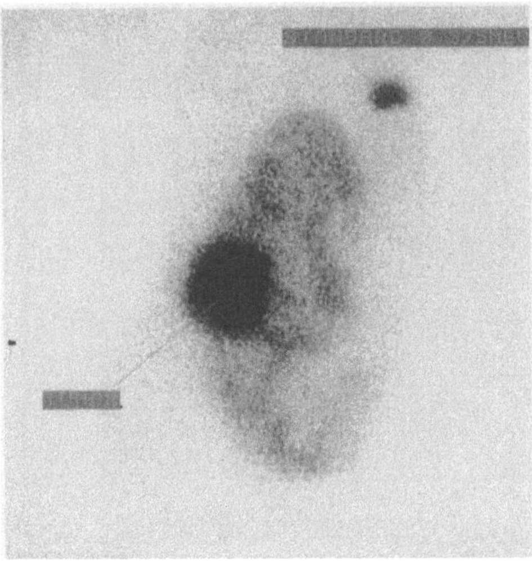

Fig. 4. Immunoscintigraphy of a clear cell carcinoma-bearing human kidney 29 h after nephrectomy (same as in Fig. 3). Enrichment of $^{99}Tc^{m}$-labeled monoclonal antibody 138H11 in the tumor is up to seven fold greater than in the remaining kidney cortex. (At the upper right a technecium standard, black, 0.3 MBq, is visible)

using mAb 138H11 and urine samples of patients with RCC (unpublished results).

Concluding Remarks

Our results indicate a possible use of mAb 138H11 for pre-, intra-, and post-surgical diagnosis and classification of primary renal tumors and metastases by the application of immunoscintigraphy, immunohistochemistry, and/or quantitative immunoassays. These applications may indicate future choices of therapy.

References

Fischer P, Scherberich JE (1989) A monoclonal antibody to gamma-glutamyltransferases of human kidneys and renal tumors. Biol Chem Hoppe Seyler 370: 620

Fischer P, Scherberich JE, Schoeppe W (1990) Comparative biochemical and immunological studies on gamma-glutamyltransferases from human kidney and renal cell carcinoma applying monoclonal antibodies. Clin Chim Acta 191: 185–200

Fischer P, Störkel S, Haase W, Scherberich JE (1991a) Monoclonal antibody 138H11 directed against gamma-glutamyl-transferase: new diagnostic and histogenetic aspects of human epithelial renal tumors. Cancer Immunol Immunother (in press)
Fischer P, Baum RP, Tauber M, Boeckmann W, Weier S, Scherberich JE (1991b) Immunoscintigraphic localization of human renal clear cell carcinomas using Technecium-99 labeled monoclonal antibody 138H11 in a human perfusion model. Cancer Res (submitted)
Hada T, Higashino K, Yamamoto H, et al. (1978) Further investigations on a novel gamma-glutamyl transpeptidase in human renal carcinoma. Clin Chim Acta 85: 267–277
Ortmann M, Vierbuchen M, Fischer R (1988) Renal oncocytoma. II. Lectin and immunohistochemical features indicating an origin from the collecting duct. Virchows Arch [B] 56: 175–184
Scherberich JE, Gauhl C, Mondorf W (1978) Biochemical, immunological and ultrastructural studies on brush-border membranes of human kidney. Curr Probl Clin Biochem 8: 85–95
Schwarz A, Steinsträsser A (1987) A novel approach to Tc-99m labeled monoclonal antibodies. J Nucl Med 28: 721
Störkel S, Jacobi GH (1989) Systematik, Histogenese und Prognose der Nierenzellkarzinome und des renalen Onkozytoms. Verh Dtsch Ges Pathol 73: 321–338
Störkel S, Pannen B, Thoenes W, Steart PV, Wagner S, Drenckhahn D (1988) Intercalated cells as a probable source for the development of renal oncocytoma. Virchows Arch [B] 56: 185–189
Störkel S, Steart PV, Drenckhahn D, Thoenes W (1989) The human chromophobe renal carcinoma: its probable relation to intercalated cells of the collecting duct. Virchows Arch [B] 56: 237–245
Taniguchi N, House S, Kuzumaki N, et al. (1985) A monoclonal antibody against gamma-glutamyltransferase from human primary hepatoma: its use in enzyme-linked immunosorbent assay of sera of cancer patients. J Natl Cancer Inst 75: 841–847
Thoenes W, Störkel S, Rumpelt HJ (1986) Histopathology and classification of renal cell tumors (adenomas, oncocytomas and carcinomas). Pathol Res Pract 181: 125–43
Toya D, Sawabu N, Ozaki K, Wakabayashi T, Nakagen M, Hattori N (1983) Purification of gamma-glutamyl transpeptidase (g-GTP) from human hepatocellular carcinoma, and comparison of g-GTP with the enzyme from human kidney. Ann N Y Acad Sci 417: 486–96
Van Dijk J, Oosterwijk E, van Kroonenburgh MJPG, et al. (1988) Perfusion of tumor-bearing kidneys as a model for scintigraphic screening of monoclonal antibodies. J Nucl Med 29: 1078–1082
Vanderlaan M, Phares W (1981) Gamma-glutamyl transpeptidase: a tumor cell marker with a pharmacological function. Histochem J 13: 865–877
Zerban H, Nogueira E, Riedasch G, Bannasch P (1987) Renal oncocytoma: origin from the collecting duct. Virchows Arch [B] 52: 375–387

T-Cell Activation by Bispecific Monoclonal Antibodies for Lysis of Renal Cell Carcinoma In Vitro

J. van Dijk[1], S.Th. Zegveld[1], J.D.H. van Eendenburg[1], E. Braakman[2], G.J. Fleuren[1], R.L.H. Bolhuis[2], and S.O. Warnaar[1]

Introduction

Patients with distant metastases from renal cell carcinoma (RCC) have a poor prognosis: The median survival is 6–8 months. Because of the relative resistance to radio- and chemotherapy, RCC patients may benefit from new treatment modalities, e.g., immunotherapy.

Because several tumor-associated antigens (TAA) are selectively expressed on tumor cells and are absent or present in low density on normal tissue, monoclonal antibodies (MAbs) reactive with these TAA may have clinical potential. In our laboratory, a number of MAbs reactive with RCC have been developed which are now being used routinely for diagnosis of RCC. One of these MAbs, G250, recognizes 96% of primary and 88% of metastatic RCC (Oosterwijk et al. 1986). For immunotherapeutic studies, we have developed bispecific MAbs by somatic hybridization of two mouse hybridomas, one producing MAbs against the T-cell antigen CD3 and the other against the G250 RCC TAA (van Dijk et al. 1989). The CD3 antigen is physically associated with the T-cell receptor (TCR) heterodimer. Binding of MAbs to the CD3/TCR complex in a crosslinked fashion results in a delivery of a signal via CD3, triggering the lytic machinery of cytotoxic T lymphocytes (CTL) (review Bolhuis et al. 1986). This MAb-mediated activation of T lymphocytes mimics the activation that physiologically occurs upon recognition of antigen by TCR. So, bispecific MAbs reactive with CD3 and G250 antigen bridge the T lymphocyte and the tumor cell and simultaneously activate the T cell

[1] University of Leiden, Department of Pathology, Wassenaarseweg 62, NL-2300 RC Leiden, The Netherlands
[2] Daniel den Hoed Cancer Center, Department of Immunology, Rotterdam, The Netherlands

G. Staehler S. Pomer (Eds.)
Basic and Clinical Research on Renal Cell Carcinoma

for lysis of the tumor cell. Furthermore bispecific antibodies were made by chemically crosslinking the OKT3 MAb, reactive with CD3 antigen, and the MRK16 MAb, reactive with P glycoprotein, overexpressed on multidrug-resistant (MDR) tumor cells (van Dijk et al. 1989). Both bispecific antibodies were tested for their ability to induce CTL to lyse RCC tumor cell lines in vitro.

Results

Induction of Tumor Cell Lysis with Bispecific MAb CD3/G250

Four different bispecific MAbs were produced by somatic hybridization of the anti-CD3 MAb producing hybridoma (IgG_{2a} isotype) with the G250 hybridoma producing different isotypes (IgG_1, IgG_{2a}, IgG_{2b}, IgE). The resulting quadromas were tested in immunohistochemistry on frozen tissue sections of RCC and spleen. In most cases no more than three cloning steps were needed to stabilize production of hybrid MAb. All stabilized quadromas with different isotype combinations (with exception of the bispecific MAb CD3/G250 (IgG_{2a}/IgE)) were able to effectively lyse the RCC target A704 using $TCR\alpha\beta^+/CD3^+$

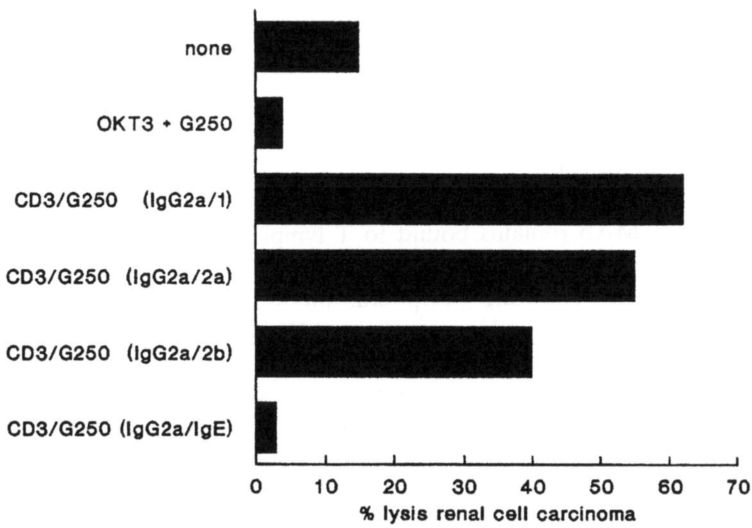

Fig. 1. Lysis of the RCC tumor cell line A704 by the $TCR\alpha\beta/CD3^+$ CTL clone D11 in the presence of bispecific MAb CD3/G250. Effector to target ratio 10:1. [1]parental MAbs

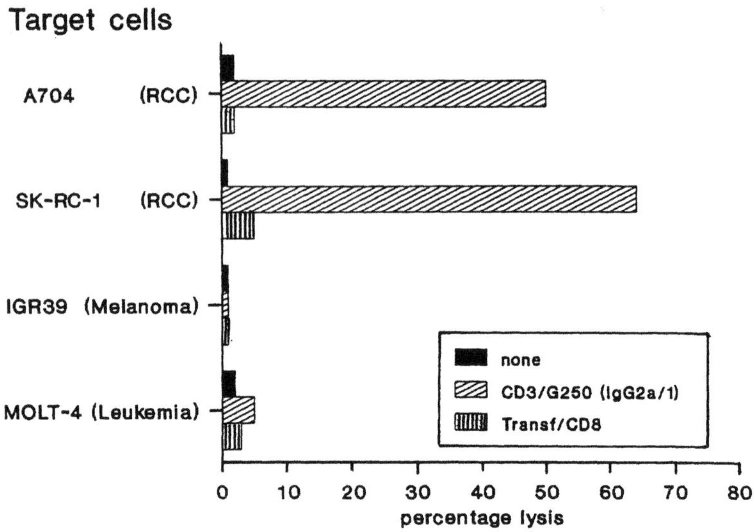

Fig. 2. Tumor cell lysis by the TCRαβ/$CD3^+$ CTL clone D11 in the presence of bispecific MAb CD3/G250 (IgG2a/1). Effector to target ratio 10:1. [1] parental MAbs

CTL clone D11. A combination of both "parental" MAbs did not induce cytolysis (Fig. 1).

As shown in Fig. 2, target cell lysis by CTL targeted with bispecific MAb CD3/G250 is selective, because two other tumor cell lines, IGR39 (melanoma) and MOLT-4 (leukemia), were not lysed. Furthermore, an irrelevant bispecific MAb Transf/CD8 did not induce lysis of tumor cells.

For possible clinical use of bispecific MAbs, it is a prerequisite that bispecific MAb remains bound to T lymphocytes sufficiently long to mediate their lytic capacity. Preincubation of $CD3^+$ T lymphocytes (activated by culturing peripheral blood lymphocytes, PBL) with phytohaemagglutin and low amounts of IL-2, 100 U/ml) with saturating amounts of bispecific MAb CD3/G250 results in tumor cell lysis, which is enhanced by additional bispecific MAb (Table 1). After 24 h, however, fluorescence-activated cell sorter (FACS) analysis of the preincubated PBL showed that considerable amounts of bispecific antibody are shed from the cell surface (data not shown), resulting in low amounts of tumor cell lysis (Table 1). However, addition of fresh bispecific MAb results in maximal tumor cell lysis, indicating that bispecific MAb is capable of binding to freshly synthesized CD3/TCR complexes.

Table 1. Lysis of RCC by activated PBL, preincubated with CD3/G250 bispecific MAb

Preincubation	MAb added during assay	% specific lysis of RCC	
		0 hr*	24 hr
–	–	5	3
–	CD3/G250	59	50
CD3/G250	–	30	8
CD3/G250	CD3/G250	50	50

PHA/IL-2 activated PBL were preincubated with either medium or CD3/G250 bispecific MAb (10 μg/ml) for 1 hr, 4°C. After washing cells were incubated at 37°C for 24 hours, and tested in a ^{51}Cr release assay in the absence or presence of soluble CD3/G250 bispecific MAb (final concentration 100 ng/ml). Target cells: RCC Scatt. Effector to target ratio 50:1

* Time of culture of CD3/G250 preincubated PBL

Biodistribution studies with ^{125}I-labeled CD3/G250 bispecific MAb in human RCC tumor-bearing nude mice clearly shows accumulation of bispecific MAb in tumor tissue with tumor to blood ratios starting from 3.4 after 6 h, increasing up to a tumor to blood ratio of 24 after 48 h, whereas no accumulation of bispecific MAb in normal tissue was observed (Fig. 3).

Induction of Tumor Cell Lysis by Bispecific Antibodies Reactive with MDR Tumor Cell Lines

Bispecific antibodies were made by chemically crosslinking OKT3 Mabs (anti-CD3) with MRK16 MAbs (anti-P glycoprotein) and tested in cytotoxicity assays for induction of lysis of MDR tumor cell lines by activated T lymphocytes. The bispecific Ab CD3/MRK16 did not mediate lysis of drug-sensitive ovarian cell line A2780 and melanoma cell line BRO. In contrast, the drug-resistant cell lines 2780AD and clone 1.1 were lysed by CTL retargeted with bispecific Ab CD3/MRK16 (Table 2). Tumor cell lines derived from RCC patients showed differences in susceptibility for lysis by retargeted CTL. FACS analysis showed that the amount of induction by CTL in the presence of bispecific Ab CD3/MRK16 was dependent on the presence or absence of P glycoprotein on the cell membrane, indicating that the

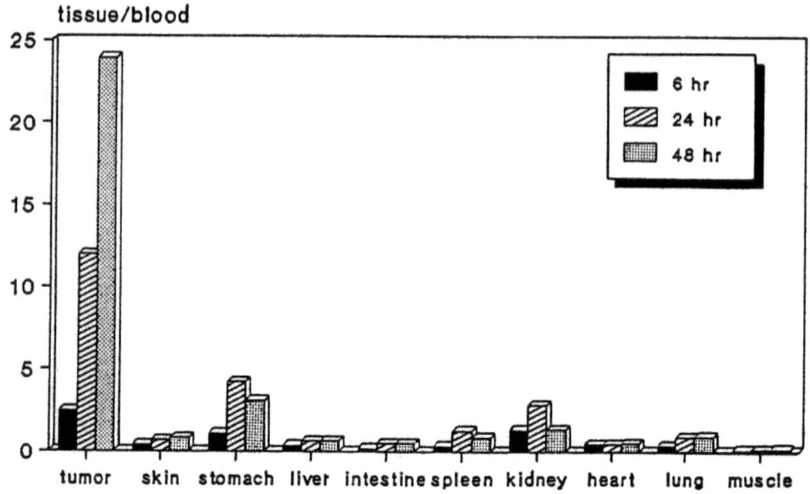

Fig. 3. In vivo biodistribution of ^{125}I-labeled bispecific MAb CD3/G250 F(ab')2 in human RCC-bearing nude mice. Mice were injected with 5 µg of MAb and were sacrificed at various time points. Tumor and normal organs were dissected, washed and weighed. Tissue to blood ratios were calculated by dividing % injected dose per gram tissue (%ID/g) by %ID/g blood

Table 2. Tumor cell lysis by cloned T lymphocytes induced by bispecific antibody CD3/MRK16

Cell line		Antibodies	
		None	bs-Ab
Ovarian	A2780	12*	10
	2780AD	45	69
Melanoma	BRO	13	10
	clone 1.1	6	35
RCC	A704	19	48
	SK-RC-6	18	36
	SK-RC-45	10	18
	SK-RC-52	1	8
	Scatt	15	15

Cloned TCRαβ/CD3* CTL D11 were tested in a ^{51}Cr release assay on various tumor cell lines in the absence or presence of bispecific antibody CD3/MRK16 (final concentration 100 ng/ml). Ovarian cell line 2780 and melanoma cell line BRO are drug sensitive, whereas 2780AD and clone 1.1 are drug resistant. Effector to target ratio 10:1

* Percentage tumor cell lysis

bispecific Ab CD3/MRK16 reacts specifically with the P glycoprotein on the various tumor cell lines.

References

Bolhuis RLH, Gravekamp C, van de Griend RJ (1986) Cell-cell interactions. Clin Immunol Allergy 6: 29

Oosterwijk E, Ruiter DJ, Hoedemaeker PhJ, Pauwels EKJ, Jonas U, Zwartendijk J, Warnaar SO (1986) Monoclonal antibody G250 recognizes a determinant present in renal cell carcinoma and absent from normal kidney. Int J Cancer 38: 489–494

van Dijk J, Warnaar SO, van Eendenburg JDH, et al. (1989) Induction of tumor cell lysis by bispecific monoclonal antibodies recognizing renal cell carcinoma and CD3 antigen. Int J Cancer 43: 344–349

van Dijk J, Tsuruo T, Segal DM, et al. (1989) Bispecific antibodies reactive with the multi-drug-resistance-related glycoprotein and CD3 induce lysis of multidrug-resistant tumor cells. Int J Cancer 44: 738–743

Immunotherapy of Renal Cell Carcinoma

New Experimental Approaches to the Adoptive Immunotherapy of Cancer: Cytokines, Gene Therapy, Oncogenes and Transgenic Mice

B.A. Fox[1]

Introduction

Adoptive immunotherapy can be defined as transfer to the tumor bearing host of active immunologic cells with antitumor reactivity that can mediate, directly or indirectly, the regression of established tumors. Within this definition there are at least two distinct approaches to this form of therapy: One is a tumor-specific approach, envisioned as mediated by a classical cytotoxic or T-helper lymphocyte, and the second is a nonspecific approach, potentially mediated by natural killer (NK) cells or a promiscuous cytotoxic T cell.

The concept of developing an autologous T cell which would specifically recognize tumor cells and selectively mediate their destruction in vitro and in vivo has fascinated and driven a community of cellular immunologists for many years. However, it was not until the revelation that interleukin (IL)-2 could be utilized as a growth factor to maintain T cells in continuous culture that rapid progress in this direction was made – similar to the onset of hybridoma technology, which allowed the humoral immunologist to generate monoclonal antibodies which recognized tumor-specific determinants. The availability of T cell growth factor (TCGF), and later recombinant IL-2, were catalysts which spurred the development of T cell lines and clones, which specifically recognized tumor cells. It was during the search for such tumor-specific T cells that a nonspecific lymphoid cell was identified. This cell was initially observed as a "contaminant" which continuously interfered with the isolation of "tumor-specific" cells. Frustrated by many attempts to generate a tumor-specific cell, Rosenberg's laboratory decided to focus on the

[1] Department of Surgery, University of Michigan Medical Center, 1520 MSRBI, Box 0666, Ann Arbor, MI 48109, USA

G. Staehler S. Pomer (Eds.)
Basic and Clinical Research on Renal Cell Carcinoma

contaminating cell population. Their analyses demonstrated that these nonspecific or lymphokine-activated killer (LAK) cells could recognize and destroy a wide variety of tumor cells and were easily generated from both mice and humans following exposure to lymphokine. Initially described as a T-cell population, subsequent studies using rIL-2 identified that LAK cells were primarily derived from NK cells. The ensuing controversy was subsequently settled when it was demonstrated that LAK generated using TCGF (which contains a wide variety of cytokines, including IL-2) was different than LAK generated in rIL-2 alone (reviewed in [6]).

In 1984 Mulé and colleagues described the capacity of LAK to mediate the regression of tumor metastases in a murine tumor model [9]. These results demonstrated that while the adoptive transfer of LAK cells alone could reduce experimentally induced metastases, concomitant administration of rIL-2 to the tumor bearing host could increase the therapeutic benefit. These findings opened the way for the pioneering clinical studies of Rosenberg which late in 1984 explored the therapeutic potential of LAK cells with concomitant administration of rIL-2. This demonstrated for the first time that it was feasible to obtain, grow and safely administer back to the patient large numbers of activated cells. While a population of patients benefited from LAK and rIL-2 therapy, it was not the panacea that some had thought it might be. Results from the clinical trials suggested that meaningful responses were observed in 20%–30% of patients who had failed conventional therapy or for whom no conventional therapy existed [13]. While these results brought calls to eliminate funding of adoptive immunotherapy trials from some corners, scientists in the field saw it as a sign that this new form of therapy could work. With increased fervor, new approaches were explored to develop cells with augmented therapeutic efficacy.

In the spring and summer of 1985 two different groups of investigaters working in Rosenberg's laboratory at the National Cancer Institute independently developed separate approaches to the generation of T cells with specific antitumor properties (Table 1). These two different experimental methods, which allowed for the generation and expansion of T cells with therapeutic properties, were; tumor-infiltrating lymphocytes (TIL), and in vitro sensitized lymphocytes (IVS) [12, 17]. Several basic aspects of these different approaches to adoptive immunotherapy are presented in Table 1. TIL were derived by simply culturing an enzymatically digested single-cell suspension of a tumor in rIL-2. After 7–10 days of culture the majority of tumor cells were eliminated and the lymphoid cells, which had represented

Table 1. Comparison of LAK, TIL and IVS

	LAK	T Cell	
		TIL	IVS
Source	PBL	Tumor	LNC
Phenotype[1]	$CD3^-$ $CD56^+$	$CD3^+$ $CD56^-$	$CD3^+$ $CD56^-$
Lytic Activity	MHC Non Restricted	MHC Restricted	MHC Restricted
Specificity of Lytic Activity[2]	Fresh Autol. and Allogeneic Tumor	Autol. Tumor	Autol. Tumor

[1] This phenotype description is a summary of the generally accepted phenotype observed for these populations. The CD3 phenotype defines a T cell population, while the CD56 phenotype defines the natural killer (NK) population.
[2] This describes the general profile of lytic activity observed for these populations. Possible target recognition repertoires include either autologous or allogeneic tumors.

less than 5% of the starting population, had rapidly expanded and now dominated the culture. These cells demonstrated some level of specific tumor recognition in vitro, as they would lyse the specific tumor line from which they were derived more efficiently than they would an unrelated tumor line (relative specificity). Most importantly, these new effector cells appeared to be 50 to 100 times more therapeutic than LAK cells on a cell-per-cell basis. These results in the animal models generated considerable enthusiasm in the laboratory, and clinical trials of TIL were initiated.

The IVS method initially utilized lymph nodes draining progressively growing tumors as the source of T cells and demonstrated that by restimulating with tumor cells in vitro, a T cell with specific therapeutic activity could be derived from the lymph node. Similar to TIL, these IVS T cells demonstrated significantly augmented therapeutic activity when compared to LAK cells. Furthermore, the IVS approach offers an alternative source of sensitized T cells for those classes of tumors from which it has been impossible to isolate or generate TIL. Recently, this approach has been modified in an attempt to better control the generation of sensitized T cells. Under this new protocol, patients are immunized with a preparation of irradiated autologous tumor cells and bacillus calmette-guérin (BCG). Ten to 14 days following immunization the draining lymph nodes are excised and cultured with autologous tumor cells and IL-2. Within 2 weeks, the cells have expanded and are infused back into the patient, together with a course of IL-2. Chang, Shu and colleagues have initiated a phase I clinical trial of IVS T cells at the University of Michigan.

Murine Tumor Models

Central to the development of these new therapies have been murine tumor models. A series of chemically induced sarcomas which were determined to be weakly immunogenic have been considered as more "relevant" to the human situation because of their weak immunogenic nature. These types of tumors are induced in mice by the intramuscular injection of 0.1% of 3-methylcholanthrene in sesame seed oil. After several months primary tumors begin to appear. These tumors are harvested, catalogued and aliquots are both cryopreserved and passaged into syngeneic mice (outlined in Fig. 1). Large numbers of tumors cells from early passages are cryopreserved and maintained as seed stocks for future studies. These tumor lines are intentionally used only in the early passages in the hope of limiting the expression of tumor heterogeneity and reducing variability inherent in these in vivo studies. The immunogenicity of these tumors is determined by demonstrating their capacity for growth in an immunized host. Those tumors which are strongly immunogenic fail to grow in an immunized animal, while those which are less immunogenic may grow in a percentage of animals tested [16]. Nonimmunogenic tumors cannot be immunized against, and therefore will always grow in immunized animals. One of the most frequently used methods of generating established tumors is the induction of experimental pulmonary metastases. These metastases are initiated by the intravenous injection of a single cell suspension of tumor. Three days later, microscopic examination of the lung has revealed that micrometastatic lesions have established in the lung. Therefore, the tumor burden in the animal is considered to be established, and treatment can be initiated. By 2 weeks following the intravenous injection, the lungs and often the liver contain numerous metastatic lesions. Animals are killed and immobilized and the lungs are insufflated with an India ink solution. Once these lungs are removed and bleached, the metastases are easily enumerated as white nodules on a black background of normal pulmonary tissue. Careful titration of the administered tumor inoculum

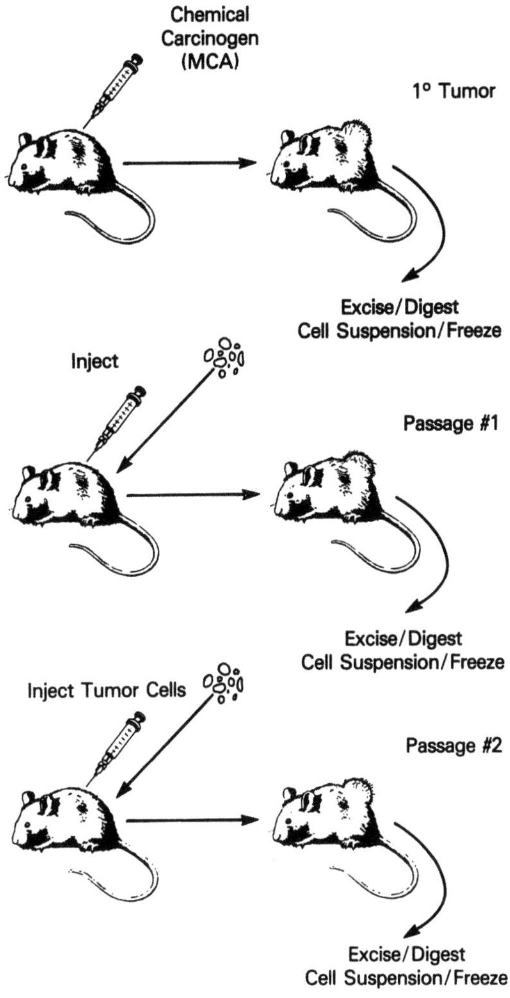

Fig. 1. In this model, primary tumors are induced by the i.m. injection of 0.1 ml of 0.1% 3-methylcholanthrene in sesame oil. Generally, the tumors which develop under these conditions appear as fibrosarcomas. These tumors are maintained in vivo in syngeneic animals by serial s.c. or i.m. transplantation of freshly isolated or cryopreserved tumor samples. When the passage number of the tumor approaches 10, it is discarded and a vial of cryopreserved tumor from an earlier passage is thawed and transplanted into syngeneic mice

can routinely generate greater than 250 metastatic lesions in the lungs of control animals. Experimental therapies can then be analyzed for their therapeutic efficacy by indexing the magnitude of tumor reduction. Modification of the host, either by radiation, cyclophosphamide, or monoclonal antibody treatment, can allow for dissection of the mechanism responsible for tumor regression. These models were instrumental in the development of strategies for LAK, TIL and IVS clinical trials. Utilizing these models LAK cells were shown to be effective mediators of tumor regression of established micrometastatic tumor. The clinical trials demonstrated, as the animal models had predicted, that LAK together with the concomitant administration of IL-2 could induce the regression of established tumor burdens in selected patients and opened the first phase of cellular immunotherapy.

Clinical Trials of TIL: Why Are the Results Not Better?

In 1986 a phase I clinical trial of TIL and IL-2 was initiated at the National Cancer Institute. While preliminary reports were encouraging, larger numbers of patients failed to respond and complete responses did not appear to be durable [14]. At face value these clinical results appeared to conflict with the animal data which suggested that TIL might be 50 to 100 times more therapeutic than LAK cells. In fact, some of these results were predicted by experience with the animal model. Based on data from the experimental models, it has been the opinion of Dr. Rosenberg's laboratory that "more is always better." In fact, almost every aspect of data seems to support that. However, to generate the large number of TIL believed necessary to mediate regression of major tumor burdens, TIL were retained in culture far longer than any TIL used in the animal studies. In retrospect it is clear from recent animal data that after 4 weeks in culture, TIL grown in high dose IL-2 (1000 μ/ml) without tumor stimulation can rapidly lose therapeutic efficacy [8]. Now Abersold and colleagues report in a summary of the in vitro parameters analyzed for the first 55 patients treated in the National Cancer Institutes TIL trial that there was a significant difference ($p2 = 0.0008$) in culture times of patients who responded to TIL therapy as compared to patients who failed to respond [1]. Furthermore, only one patient whose cells were cultured more than 42 days responded. This data can arguably be interpreted as supporting the hypothesis, derived from the animal experience, that TIL cultured in high dose IL-2 (1000 U/ml) lose therapeutic efficacy with time in culture.

Recently we have demonstrated that therapeutic efficacy can be maintained in clones of T cells derived from TIL by routine stimulation with tumor cells and culture in a relatively low dose of IL-2 (25 μ/ml) [8]. We have observed similar results with bulk TIL cultures grown in the lower dose of IL-2 and repeatedly stimulated with tumor cells every 10 to 14 days (unpublished observation). Thus is appears that therapeutic efficacy can be maintained by regulating culture conditions in animal models. Can this approach of utilizing routine tumor stimulation and culture in low dose IL-2 be employed in a clinical protocol? In general it appears unlikely, since it is often difficult to recover from patients the large numbers of viable tumor cells required for a protocol of this nature. This roadblock to the expansion of therapeutic cells has at least two possible alternatives. The first is to substitute cultured tumor cells as a source of stimulator cells in vitro. At least for melanoma tumors, this may be a viable option as these cells can routinely be cultured and expanded in vitro. Further, with the recent proposal that there may be a common melanoma antigen it is possible that a bank of melanoma tissue culture lines of known histocompatibility locus antigen (HLA) haplotypes may serve as a reservoir of stimulator cells, which could be drawn upon as needed [5]. These tumors would not have to be perfect matches. In fact they may only have to share a single HLA class I antigen. In the case of HLA-A2 for example, information from the Eighth International HLA Workshop suggests that it is shared by 46.6% of North American Caucasians and 45.3% of European Caucasians. Thus a single tumor line might possibly serve as a stimulator line for over 40% of melanoma patients presenting for therapy.

Alternatively, primed T cells may be triggered by a monoclonal antibody to the CD3 antigen or to the T cell receptor (TCR). Such triggering, occurring through the recognition/transducing structure on the T cell may mimic the physiologic stimulation of a tumor cell. Recently Yoshizawa and collaborators in Shu's laboratory documented that such an approach was effective in triggering the maturation of tumor sensitized but nonfunctional pre-effector cells into therapeutic effector cells. Cells triggered in this fashion were able to mediate regression of pulmonary metastases and cure animals with advanced tumor burdens [20]. These results provide a rationale for triggering and/or expanding autologous sensitized T cells for the treatment of patients with cancer.

Immunotherapy with Cytokines

Two predictions from the animal model which are relevant to immunotherapy with cytokines alone are:

1. Tumor cell expression of major histocompatibility complex (MHC) class I antigen correlates with the tumors susceptibility to cytokine treatment in vivo.
2. The capacity to grow $CD8^+$ T cells from the tumor in vitro correlates with the tumors susceptibility to cytokine treatment in vivo.

Both of these predictions are based upon observations made in animal models in which a $CD8^+$ effector alone appears to be the effective mediator of tumor destruction. These generalizations could foreseeably be expanded to include expression of MHC class II antigen, if a $CD4^+$ effector could be identified. These predictions appear consistent within the methylcholanthrene (MCA)-induced tumor model (MCA 101, 102, 105, and 106) for the following cytokines; IL-2, interferon (IFN)γ, IFNα, and tumor necrosis factor (TNF)α. Experiments were performed using four different MCA tumors, two which are weakly immunogenic (MCA 105 and 106) and two which are apparently nonimmunogenic (MCA 101 and 102). Utilizing these tumors in the model system defined above, a distinction could be drawn between immunogenic and nonimmunogenic tumors and for micrometastatic and macrometastatic tumor burdens.

Micrometastatic disease is defined in this system as the tumor burden which is established 3–4 days following intravenous or intrasplenic injection of tumor cells. Untreated, this level of tumor burden will grow progressively and kill the recipient in 2–3 weeks. Macrometastatic diseae is generally defined as the level of tumor burden existing 10–14 days following the intravenous/intrasplenic injection of tumor cells. Animals killed at this time have clearly visible metastatic lesions on the surface of the lung and or liver. Utilizing these designations of micrometastatic or macrometastatic disease, a further delineation of antitumor activity can be ascribed to the cytokines or cells tested.

The data presented in Table 2 is a summary of many experiments performed by investigators in Rosenberg's laboratory. The mechanism of cytokine-induced regression is best understood for IL-2. Mulé et al. performed an elegant series of experiments which clearly dissected the mechanism of IL-2-induced regression of pulmonary metastases [10]. Those experiments, summarized in part of Table 2, demonstrated that the IL-2-induced regression of 3-day pulmonary

Table 2. Effect of cytokine treatment on experimental metastases

Cytokine treatment	Day 3 micrometastases[1]		Day 10 macrometastases[2]	
	MCA 101/102 MHC class I^-	MCA 105/106 MHC class I^+	MCA 101/102 MHC class I^-	MCA 105/106 MHC class I^+
IL-2	+	+	–	+
(mediated by)	(LAK)	(LAK^+ & $CD8^+$)	(–)	($CD8^+$)
IFNα	–	+	–	–
IL-2 + IFNα	+	+	+/–	++
IFNγ	ND	ND	ND	–
IL-2 + IFNγ	ND	ND	ND	+/++
IL-4	ND	–	ND	ND
IL-4 + IL-2	ND	+/++	ND	ND
IL-6	ND	+	ND	ND

[1] Day 3 micrometastases were induced as described in the section on murine tumor models. Metastases were induced with either of the MCA tumors listed.
[2] Day 10 macrometastases were induced as above, utilizing the tumors identified.

metastases were mediated by LAK cells for the nonimmunogenic MCA-102 tumor and mediated by both CD8$^+$ and LAK cells for the weakly immunogenic MCA-106 tumor. However, when advanced macrometastatic disease was treated with IL-2, the nonimmunogenic tumor did not regress and the regression of the weakly immunogenic tumor was mediated solely by a CD8$^+$ T cell. These data suggests that:

1. in vivo generated LAK cells fail to impact on advanced tumor burdens,
2. CD8$^+$ T cells fail to contribute to regression of the nonimmunogenic MCA tumors; and
3. only CD8$^+$ T cells are effective at mediating the regression of advanced tumor burdens in this model.

Furthermore, extrapolation of this data to clinical trials might suggest that regression of large tumor burdens is a function of resident CD8$^+$ T cells (TIL), and not a function of adoptively transferred LAK.

The addition of IFNα or IFNγ to IL-2 in this model appears to be synergistic only for the weakly immunogenic tumor where a CD8$^+$ T cell is mediating tumor regression. These studies performed by Cameron and colleagus further demonstrated that the synergistic effect of these cytokines was dependent on a radiosensitive host component (Table 2) [4]. If one accepts the premise that the weakly immunogenic tumors are eliminated by a CD8$^+$ T cell which recognizes an antigenic determinant in the context of the MHC class I molecule present on the tumor cells membrane, and that it takes 7–10 days to generate a primary cellular response, then it would seem likely that treatment of a tumor-bearing recipient on day 10, with a cytokine (like IFN) which upregulates class I expression, would not leave sufficient time for an immune response to be evoked. Since, by the time 7–10 days more had elapsed, enough time to generate an immune response, the animal would have died of metastatic disease. An alternative experimental design would be to begin treating nonimmunogenic micrometastases on day 3 with IFNγ or IFNα, at doses which have been shown to upregulate MHC class I expression. Then by day 10, when advanced metastases have developed, initiate treatment with IL-2 alone. Hypothetically, such a protocol would induce class I expression, which would allow for the induction of an immune response by day 10. Initiation of IL-2 therapy at that time might then allow for the expansion of a CD8$^+$ T cell with therapeutic activity.

TNFα is a cytokine that possesses significant antitumor properties both in vitro and in vivo. A single i.v. dose of this cytokine can mediate regression of large subcutaneous tumor burdens for tumors with demonstrated immunogenicity. Regression of these subcutaneous tumor burdens requires $CD8^+$, but not $CD4^+$ T cells [2]. Tumors which are nonimmunogenic can undergo hemorrhagic necrosis, but do not regress. Unfortunately, TNF has not demonstrated an anti-tumor effect against either experimentally induced micrometastatic or macrometastatic tumor burdens. Furthermore, studies combining TNF with IL-2 have not revealed any synergistic activity in the treatment of weakly immunogenic pulmonary metastases (J. McIntosh and J. Mulé, unpublished observation). Future studies need to address the potential role of TNF in the development of cytokine combinations which may be more effective in the treatment of both micrometastatic and macrometastatic lesions.

Coupling Combination Cytokine Therapy with Adoptive Transfer of T Cells

The previous experiments were directed at synergizing exogenously administered cytokines with the endogenous host component to mediate regression of established tumor, realizing that there were a number of possible antagonizing factors in the tumor-bearing mouse. We next investigated whether additional cytokines could augment the therapeutic efficacy of adoptively transferred effector cells. A series of studies were initiated utilizing a T-cell clone of TIL derived from a murine colon adenocarcinoma (MC-38). This T-cell clone, BF-1, expressed the phenotypic characteristics listed in Table 3 and was

Table 3. Flow microfluorometric analysis of the BF-1 T cell clone

Monoclonal antibody	Antigenic determinant	% Cells positive
53–67	CD 8	90.4
GK1.5	CD 4	2.6
2.4G2	Fc receptor	2.4
2C11	CD 3	69.3
6C7	LY 6	84.6
D7	LY 6	93.3
M5114	Ia	9.1
B220	B cell	6.7
M19	CLA	93.5
7D4	IL-2 receptor	26.7
3C7	IL-2 receptor	28.0
211	Human T/NK cells	3.5

maintained in continuous culture with a low dose of IL-2 (25 U/ml) and repeated tumor stimulation. A cultured line of the MC-38 tumor was utilized for repetitive stimulation (to decrease incidence of contamination) and also employed as a target for in vitro cytotoxicity assays. Generally, the BF-1 T-cell clone exhibited a pattern of absolute specificity, efficiently lysing the MC-38 tumor of origin without killing either unrelated syngeneic tumor targets or YAC (an NK-susceptible target cell) [8]. During this cycle of continuous culture, it became apparent that the cultured MC-38 tumor line was not always lysed as efficiently as it had been. Consideration was given to the possibility that the T-cell clone was losing some functional activity. Alternatively, the continuously cultured tumor cell line might have modified its expression of recognition structures, thereby eluding recognition and destruction. Realizing that cytokines can upregulate expression of recognition structures, tumor antigens and MHC molecules, the effect of treating MC-38 tumor targets with cytokines was examined. The cultured tumor cell line was exposed to 1000 μ/ml of IFNγ, IFNα, TNFα, IFNα + IFNγ, or IFNγ + TNFα. The effect of these cytokines on cell doubling time, viability, cell yield, "leakiness" and expression of MHC class I molecules are presented in Table 4. While there were striking differences in the uptake of ^{51}Cr label and the inherent "leakiness" of the targets, demonstrated by increased levels of spontaneous ^{51}Cr release, LAK effectors uniformly lysed all targets equally (Fig. 2, top). Contrariwise, the BF-1 effector lysed the TNFα or IFNγ + TNFα treated targets strikingly better than the nontreated control, with the targets treated with the combination of IFNγ and TNFα being lysed most effectively (Fig. 2, bottom). Analysis of MHC class I expression revealed that the nontreated MC-38 tumor cells constitutively expressed a high level of this surface molecule and cytokine-induced alterations in this level did not correlate with increased susceptibility to lysis (Table 4), therefore suggesting that another accessory or recognition structure may be responsible for this increased level of effector cell mediated destruction.

Armed with the observation that the combination of IFNγ and TNFα could modify the MC-38 tumor in such a way that it was more readily recognized or destroyed in vitro, we explored the effect of combining IFNγ and TNFα or IFNα and TNFα with the BF-1 T cell clone and IL-2 administration for the treatment of experimental pulmonary metastases. Table 5 presents a summary of data from three experiments in which IFNγ and TNFα or IFNα and TNFα were combined with BF-1 T cells and IL-2. Mice were administered 500 R prior to induction of experimental metastases and treatment was initiated

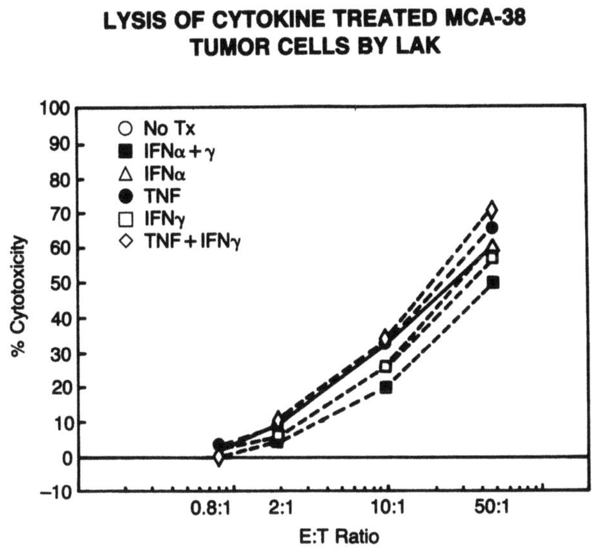

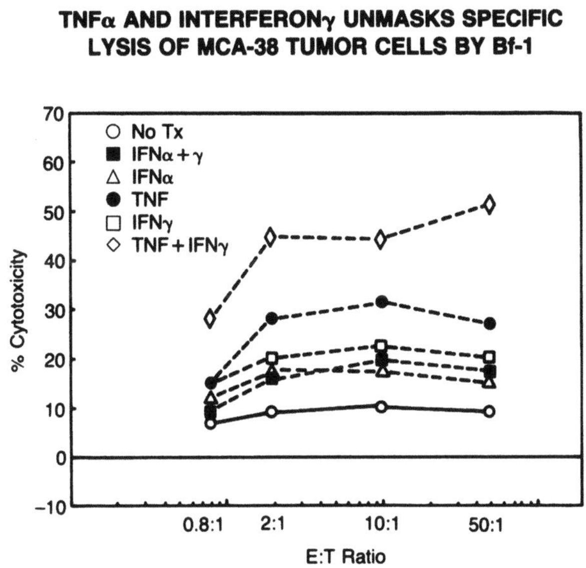

Fig. 2. LAK lysis of MC-38 tumor targets in a 4-h ^{51}Cr release assay (*top graph*). Tumor targets were cultured with the cytokines listed for 72 h prior to analysis of lysability. Control target cells were cultured in medium alone (No Tx). These same targets were analyzed for lysability by the BF-1 T cell clone (*bottom graph*)

Table 4. Effect of cytokines on cultured MCA-38 tumor cells

Treatment[1]	Yield[2] $\times 10^6$	Cell Doublings[3]	% Viable	% Control Yield	% Spontaneous Release[4] (window) cpm	MHC Class I expression[5] MCF
No TX	8.5	2+	96	100	12.8 (8747)	354
IFNγ 1000 U/ML	8.55	2+	92	100.5	15.8 (8867)	372
IFNα 1000 U/ML	4.5	1+	92	52.9	14.3 (7741)	393
TNFα 1000 U/ML	6.0	1+	88	71.4	31.1 (8733)	321
IFNα + IFNγ 1000 U/ML	6.6	2+	90	77.6	16.5 (11772)	348
IFNγ + TNFα 1000 U/ML	5.8	1+	84	68.7	32.4 (5712)	407

[1] MCA-38 tumor cells were cultured 2 days in complete medium (No Tx), or complete medium containing the cytokine listed.
[2] Number of cells recovered following 3 days of culture.
[3] Mean number of cell doublings occurring during culture.
[4] That percentage of ^{51}Cr released by control tumor cells during the 4-h cytotoxicity assay divided by the total ^{51}Cr bound by the tumor cell, multiplied by 100.
[5] Mean channel fluoresence (MCF) of MHC class I molecules determined by flow cytometry.

Table 5. Combinations of cytokines can synergize with the adoptive transfer of T cells to increase therapeutic efficacy

Adoptive Transfer[3]	Percent Reduction of Control Pulmonary Metastases[1]		
	Cytokines Administered[2]		
	IL-2	IFNγ + TNFα + IL-2	IFNα + TNFα + IL-2
None	0	28.3 ± 19	70.8 ± 21.2
BF-1 (1X)	2.4 ± 8.7	89.2 ± 3.2	91 ± 10.8
BF-1 (10X)	57.4 ± 27	99 ± 0.2	93.5 ± 8.9

[1] Percent reduction (mean ± standard deviation) was determined according to the formula;

$$\frac{\text{number of metastases in experimental group}}{\text{number of metastases in control group}} \times 100 = \%\ \text{reduction.}$$

[2] 10000 U of rIL-2 twice a day on days 3–8, 40000 U (2 experiments) of IFNγ twice a day on days 3–4 and once a day on days 5–8 (2 experiments) or 50000 U of IFNγ once a day on days 3–6 (1 experiment). 1 µg of rhTNFα once each day on days 3–8. 50000 U of IFNα twice each day for 3 days, and once a day for 3 additional days. Experimental determinations are the result of 3 determinations each, except for the BF-1 (1X) IFNγ + TNFα + IL-2, which is the result of only 2 determinations.

[3] BF-1 cells were transferred in graded doses to mice bearing experimentally induced metastases of MC-38 tumor. The 1X dosage of transferred cells ranged from 0.4–1.0 × 10^6. The 10X dosage of transferred T cells was ten fold higher than the 1X dosage (0.4–1.0 × 10^7).

on day 3. The number of metastases in control IL-2 treated mice ranged from 229 to 308. The 1X dose of BF-1 T cells ranged from 0.4–1 × 10^6 cells/recipient in different experiments. The 10X dose of BF-1 T cells was ten fold higher than the 1X dose (0.4 to 10^7 cells/recipient). Treatment of established metastases with the 1X dose of BF-1 T cells and IL-2 had no therapeutic effect, reducing the number of metastases by only 2.4%. However, a ten fold higher dosage of BF-1 T cells combined with IL-2 reduced pulmonary metastases by a mean of 57.4%. The addition of IFNγ, TNFα and IL-2, which had a minimal effect alone (28.3% reduction), to BF-1 T cells increased the therapeutic effect, reducing pulmonary metastases by 89.2% for the 1X dosage and 99% for the 10X dosage. The combination of IFNα, TNFα and IL-2 had significant antitumor activity alone, reducing the number of metastases in animals which did not receive T cells by 70.8%. The fact that this reduction is seen in sublethally irradiated animals which have not received effector T cells suggests that this cytokine combination may be mediating an effect which is independent of a lymphoid component. The addition of BF-1 T cells to this combination of cytokines demonstrated a further reduction in the number of pulmonary metastases to 91% and 93.5%, respectively, for the 1X and 10X dosage BF-1 T cells.

These data suggest that combinations of cytokines which are ineffective alone (IFNγ and TNFα) may work synergistically with adoptively transferred T cells, elaborating an antitumor effect from a suboptimal number (1X dosage) of effector cells. Furthermore, the substantial antitumor effect observed with the combination of IFNα, TNFα and IL-2 could be improved by the addition of effector cells to this therapeutic strategy. The mechanism responsible for this effect in irradiated animals is unknown. The studies of Cameron and colleagues demonstrated that IFNα combined with IL-2 did not mediate regression of micrometastatic lesions in irradiated recipients; however, it may be surmised from the data in Table 4 that both IFNα and TNFα have substantial antiproliferative activity against the MC-38 tumor cells used in these studies. Potentially, the combination of these cytokines may effectively impact on tumor burdens against which either agent used alone (or combined with IL-2) may be ineffective. Certainly, the exciting clinical approach of Otto and colleagues presented at this symposium is aimed at identifying whether the combination of IFNα and TNFα may have increased therapeutic potential compared to either agent used alone.

Immunologic Strategies for Nonimmunogenic(?) Human Tumors

As is has been difficult to identify an immune response to most classes of human tumors it has been surmised that they are predominantly nonimmunogenic. This has been a principle point of concern for the future of immunotherapy. Scientists and clinicians alike are left facing the conclusion that the capacity to grow $CD8^+$ T cells from the tumor in vitro correlates with tumor susceptibility to cytokine treatment, presumably via the induction of the same $CD8^+$ T cells in vivo. The question is therefore raised of how a T cell with antitumor activity is generated from a host bearing an apparently nonimmunogenic tumor?

Retreating to the animal model once again, Shu and colleagues documented that utilizing a tumor vaccine approach, it was possible to generate a therapeutic effector cell from the MCA 102 tumor, previously defined as nonimmunogenic [18]. Had the tumor cell line changed? Had a mutation rendered it immunogenic? Repeat analysis of its immunogenicity revealed that the tumor had retained its nonimmunogenic characteristics; however, modification of the tumor preparation had allowed for the generation of T cells with antitumor properties [18].

Next, Yang and collaborators utilized a magnetic sphere (or bead) coated with an anti-T cell antibody to purify, concentrate and stimulate TIL derived from the MCA-102 tumor [19]. These "beaded TIL" (named for the microscopic appearance of the magnetic spheres as they collect or bead around the T cells recognized by the antibody coated to the bead) also expressed therapeutic activity against the nonimmunogenic MCA-102 tumor. These two approaches suggest that manipulation of the tumor may allow for the generation of a T cell with antitumor activity from a host bearing an apparently nonimmunogenic tumor.

Applications of Gene Transfer to Adoptive Immunotherapy

Genetic engineering is a new approach to understanding and augmenting the antitumor activity of T cells. Gene therapy has been defined as a proposed therapeutic technique, in which a functioning gene is inserted into the somatic cell of a patient, to correct an inborn genetic error or to provide a new function to cells. While there are several approaches to integrate new genetic information into a cell, retroviral mediated gene transfer has several advantages. The most significant in the clinical setting may be that it is highly effective, commonly resulting in 20%–30% of cells integrating the new gene. Previously described as infection, this method has been renamed transduction (with the term infection being replaced, just as the word nuclear was replaced in nuclear magnetic resonance). Therefore we speak of transducing someone's T cells, not infecting them, with a retrovirus. Retroviral transduction of a cell is accomplished by culturing that cell with a replication defective retrovirus vector (Fig. 3). This vector for new genetic information is created by deleting a substantial portion of the retroviral genome. This includes the sequences which encode the *gag*, *pol* and *env* genes. The selected new genetic information together with some selectable marker gene and promoters are then inserted into the remaining retroviral backbone. This new genetic information is then encapsulated with a retroviral envelope provided by a producer cell. The resulting retroviral vector is capable of transducing (infecting) only once as it does not contain the re-

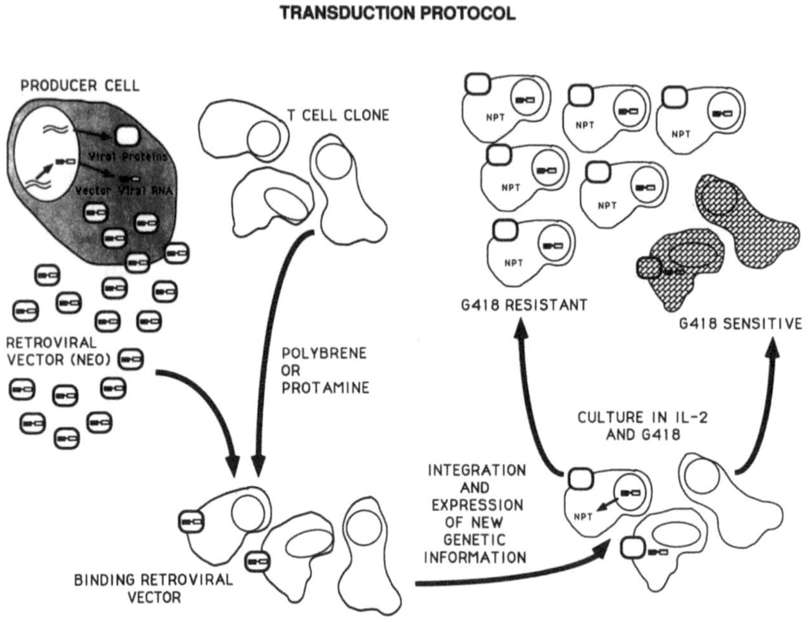

Fig. 3. Schematic model of retroviral mediated gene transfer into a T-cell clone. The producer cell secretes the replication-defective retroviral vector into the culture supernatant. This supernatant is collected, tested for competent retrovirus, and added to a culture of T cells in the presence of polybrene or protamine. If a membrane receptor is present, the vector may bind to the cell. Integration into the DNA of the new genetic information may lead to expression of that information. Cells with expression of the selectable marker gene (NPT) may be isolated and expanded in the presence of the appropriate selecting agent (G418). Cells which fail to integrate or express the selectable marker gene will die in the presence of the selecting agent

quired genetic information to replicate itself. The incorporation of a functional marker, such as the neomycin resistance gene (Neo^r), allows for the selection of cells transduced with this gene by culturing them in the neomycin analog G418. Cells which express the Neo^r gene product are able to grow in G418, while cells which lack the gene product die.

An outline of two distinct approaches to the "design of more effective T cells" are presented in Table 6. The first is an indirect approach, as the induced modification of the transduced T cell (integration of the Neo^r gene) does not confer an enhanced antitumor property. Yet this capacity to select transduced T cells by way of a newly inserted functional gene affords a novel approach to study trafficking of adop-

Table 6. Design more effective T cell populations

Indirect:
Transduce T cells with the Neo^r gene; expand populations of T cells which traffic to tumor by exploiting their capacity to grow in the neomycin analog (G418).
1. Study phenotype and characteristics of cells isolated from regressing and progressing lesions.
2. Expand, select and reinfuse T cells isolated from regressing lesions.

Direct:
Modify T cells by Gene Therapy
1. Engineer cytokine genes into T cells.
2. Customize T cells with new TCR or Ig genes.
3. Enhance lytic/effector mechanism. (perforin/esterase genes)

tively transferred T cells in the tumor-bearing host. Hypothetically, one could use this technique to transduce a heterogeneous population of T cells (either TIL or IVS) prior to reinfusion into the patient. During the follow-up period, lesions from responder and nonresponder patients could be biopsied and lymphocytes present in the biopsy could be expanded in IL-2 and selected in G418. The phenotype and functional characteristics of cells present in the responder and non-responder lesions could be analyzed and potentially a correlation drawn, which might implicate a given "type(s)" of T cell(s) as the mediator of tumor regression in vivo. Such information might allow for the selective expansion of the appropriate cell type, thereby increasing the effectiveness of treatment while potentially reducing the volume of media and reagents used. Alternatively, transduced T cells obtained from regressing lesions might be enriched for therapeutic cells and could be expanded and reinfused to the patient. Such an approach might be seen as indirectly increasing the effectiveness of the T cell.

To test our capacity to perform these trafficking studies the BF-1 T cell clone was transduced with the Neo^r gene paired with the human adenosine deaminase (huADA) gene. This transduced T cell clone maintained its pattern of specific in vitro cytotoxicity and some level of therapeutic efficacy for a time. Most importantly we were able to demonstrate to ourselves and the regulatory committee overseeing the application of this technology to the clinic (the Recombinant DNA Advisory Committee or RAC) that utilizing polymerase chain reaction (PCR), one could identify the trafficking of transduced BF-1 T cells to organs of tumor-bearing mice. Subsequently it was dem-

Table 7. The design of more effective T cells utilizing gene transfer: application of the indirect approach to IVS clinical protocol

1. Label IVS cells with the retroviral vector LNL6 or G1Na which contains the gene for neomycin resistance.
2. Reinfuse the transduced IVS cells at the time of standard IVS therapy.
3. Biopsy tumor nodules and other tissues at intervals and measure vector presence by detecting the inserted gene.
4. Culture the biopsy specimen under conditions favoring IVS growth (i.e., IL-2 plus selection with G418) to recover the infused gene marked IVS cells for analysis of phenotypic characteristics and correlation with response to treatment.
5. Expand and reinfuse T cells isolated from tumor lesions which regressed following adoptive transfer of IVS cells.

onstrated that we could recover, expand and select the transduced cells from the blood of recipient animals, and that they continued to produce both gene products (Neo^r and ADA) [7]. Based on these data from Dr. Rosenberg's laboratory, and a large experience from Anderson's and Blaese's laboratories demonstrating no toxicity in primates and the absence of any competent retrovirus contaminating the retroviral vectors, the first gene transfer protocol in humans was approved [15].

Alternatively, gene transfer affords the capability to modify T cells by the insertion of a gene which might directly augment their antitumor property. Three modifications which have the potential to accomplish this goal are listed in Table 7. The integration of genes, which encode cytokines with inherent antitumor properties, into T cells, is an aproach which is being aggressively pursued by Rosenberg, Anderson, Blaese and colleagues at the National Institutes of Health (NIH). This concept of using T cells as vehicles to deliver substances with antitumor properties to metastatic lesions has developed around the observation from Rosenberg's group that TIL can preferentially

Table 8. Potential advantages of cell-delivered cytokines

1. Transduced T cells might specifically traffic to the tumor site.
2. Specific trafficking could result in an increased concentration of cytokine at the local (tumor) site.
3. Membrane bound cytokines may have antitumor properties without the toxicity associated with a systemically administered cytokine.
4. The infused T cells and associated toxicity will be regulated by IL-2 administration.

traffic to tumor sites. Potential advantages of such an approach are itemized in Table 8. In studies which were initiated at the NIH and are being continued at the University of Michigan, in collaboration with Drs. Culver, Blaese, and Moen, we are exploring the plausibility of such an approach in animal models. Utilizing the BF-1 T cell clone as a model of T cell–tumor interaction, we have integrated the gene for human TNFα or human IL-1β into this T cell. Preliminary analyses of these novel T cells have identified highly augmented in vitro cytotoxic activity mediated by the IL-1β transduced cells. Initial studies of the BF-1 T cell clone transduced with the TNFα gene have not identified any augmentation of in vitro properties. Studies of the therapeutic potential as well as the toxicity of these novel T cells, that secrete TNFα or IL-1β, are in progress.

The concept of "customizing" T cells with alternative recognition structures is currently within reach (Table 6). Genes which encode a TCR or an immunoglobulin, with specificity for a class of tumors, could be inserted into T cells from patients with cancer. While TCR genes would have to be matched for at least one HLA class I antigen, the integration of a membrane bound immunoglobulin would not be so restricted. It might be envisioned that nonspecific T cells, expanded from the peripheral blood of patients with colon cancer, would be transduced with the gene encoding the immunoglobulin-recognizing carcinoembryonic antigen (CEA). The inserted gene would be modified such that it would remain membrane bound and could serve as a recognition and triggering structure for the transduced T cells. Such an approach may afford a technique to take advantage of immunoglobulins which recognize tumor-specific determinants to aid the trafficking, recognition, and destruction of cancer in humans.

A third approach to directly modify T cells is to enhance the effector mechanism of the T cell, by increasing the level or expression of lytic or effector molecules (Table 6). The identification of molecules associated with the lytic pathway (i.e., perforin or esterase) allows for the insertion of such into a tumor specific T cell. Hypothetically, these T cells would retain their specific recognition patterns but would become more effective mediators of tumor destruction, as a result of an increased number of effector molecules. Such approaches to the treatment of cancer must rely upon animal models to develop and test these experimental strategies. However, many of the available models may have limited application in the development of some tumor specific strategies. The development of transgenic mice, discussed below, may offer exciting alternatives to the arsenal of animal tumor models currently available.

Oncogenes and Transgenic Mice

Over the past 10 years, activated-oncogene expression has been increasingly associated with malignant transformation of tissue culture cells. Molecular analysis identified that "activation" of *ras* oncogenes routinely occurred as a result of a single specific point mutation in the structural gene. This information led to the search for, and discovery of, activated-oncogene expression in a wide variety of human neoplastic and preneoplastic tissues (reviewed in [3]). To date almost 60 oncogenes have been described and treatment strategies are being developed which may exploit the oncogene's mechanism of action. With this in mind, the concept that a single oncogenic protein/peptide may be expressed by a wide variety of tumors offers exciting and challenging prospects for tumor immunology.

The development of transgenic mouse technology has allowed for the stable integration of a particular gene construct into the host's genome. Appropriate engineering of the foreign gene construct to be inserted can target preferential expression of that gene in a particular tissue or organ. The engineering of transgenic mice with constructs containing either v-Ha-ras, c-myc, or c-neu oncogenes has led in some instances to preferential expression of oncogenes in the mammary tissue. Preferential expression of oncogenes in this tissues is, presumably, partially responsible for the high incidence of mammary adenocarcinoma observed in the v-Ha-*ras* transgenic mice. These transgenic mice develop tumors in a predictable stochastic fashion which suggests a second (unknown) factor is required for progression to the malignant state. This second factor is presumably some environmental or developmental factor. The tumors arise in an apparent clonal fashion with distinctive histologic heterogeneity between some tumors. These tumors can be locally invasive and can spontaneously metastasize to the liver and/or lung [11]. These new transgenic mouse tumor models offer the potential to study the immunobiology of a series of tumors which were "predisposed" by a single activation-specific mutation to an oncogene. The potential utility of this novel clinically relevant tumor system to the study of tumor immunobiology is obvious.

Acknowledgements. The author wishes to gratefully acknowledge the support and scientific stimulation of his mentor, Dr. Steven A. Rosenberg, who's untiring energy and creative genuis inspired and directed the majority of work reviewed in this manuscript. The helpful discussions with Drs Michael Blaese, W. French Anderson, Ken

Culver, Jim Mule', Suyu Shu and Alfred Chang and the excellent editorial assistance of Debbie Birdsall are graciously noted. Supported in part by a grant from the University of Michigan Cancer Center's Institutional Grant from the American Cancer Society.

References

1. Aebersold P, Hyatt C, Johnson S, et al. (1991) Lysis of autologous melanoma cells by tumor infiltrating lymphocytes is associated with clinical response. J Natl Cancer Inst 83: 932
2. Asher AL, Mulé JJ, Rosenberg SA (1989) Recombinant human tumor necrosis factor mediates regression of murine sarcoma in vivo via Lyt-2^+ cells. Cancer Immunol Immunother 28: 153–156
3. Bos JL (1989) *Ras* oncogenes in human cancer: A review. Cancer Research 49: 4682
4. Cameron RB, McIntosh JK, Rosenberg SA (1988) Synergistic antitumor effects of combination immunotherapy with recombinant interleukin-2 and a recombinant hybrid α-interferon in the treatment of established murine hepatic metastases. Cancer Res 48: 5810
5. Darrow TL, Singluff CL, Siegler HF (1989) The role of HLA class I antigens in recognition of melanoma cells by tumor-specific cytotoxic T lymphocytes: evidence for shared tumor antigens. J Immunol 149: 3329
6. Fox BA, Rosenberg SA (1989) Heterogeneous lymphokine-activated killer cell precursor populations; development of a monoclonal antibody that separates two populations of precursors with distinct culture requirements and separate target-recognition repertoires. Cancer Immunol Immunother 29: 155
7. Fox BA, Culver KW, Cornetta K, et al. (1989) Retroviral gene transduction of murine tumor infiltrating lymphocytes: a new approach to study trafficking in vivo. FASEB J 3: (3)3496
8. Fox BA, Spiess PJ, Kasid A, Puri RK, Mule JJ, Weber JS, Rosenberg SA (1990) In vitro and in vivo antitumor properties of a T-cell clone generated from murine tumor infiltrating lymphocytes. J Biol Response Mod 9 (5): 499
9. Mulé JJ, Shu S, Schwartz SL, et al. (1984) Successful adoptive immunotherapy of established metastases with LAK cells and recombinant interleukin 2. Science 225: 1487
10. Mulé JJ, Yang JC, Lafreniere RL, Shu SY, Rosenberg SA (1987) Identification of cellular mechanisms operational in vivo during the regression of established pulmonary metastases by the systemic administration of high-dose recombinant interleukin 2. J Immunol 7:1; 139 (1): 285
11. Pattengale PK, Stewart TA, Leder A, et al. (1989) Am J Pathol 135: 39
12. Rosenberg SA, Spiess PJ, Lafreniere R (1986) A new approach to the adoptive immunotherapy of cancer with tumor-infiltrating lymphocytes. Science 233: 1318

13. Rosenberg SA, Lotze MT, Muul LM, et al. (1987) A progress report on the treatment of 157 patients with advanced cancer using lymphokine-activated killer cells and interleukin-2 or high dose interleukin-2 alone. N Engl J Med 316: 889
14. Rosenberg SA, Packard BS, Aebersold PM (1988) Special report: use of tumor-infiltrating lymphocytes and interleukin-2 in the immunotherapy of patients with metastatic melanoma. A preliminary report. N Engl J Med 319: 1676
15. Rosenberg SA, Aebersold P, Cornetta K, et al. (1990) Gene transfer into humans – immunotherapy of patients with advanced melanoma, using tumor-infiltrating lymphocytes modified by retroviral gene transduction. N Engl J Med 323: 570
16. Shu S, Rosenberg SA (1985) Adoptive immunotherapy of newly-induced murine sarcomas. Cancer Res 45: 1657
17. Shu S, Chou T, Rosenberg SA (1986) In vitro sensitization and expansion with viable tumor cells and interleukin 2 in the generation of specific therapeutic effector cells. J Immunol 136: 3891
18. Shu S, Chou T, Sakai K (1989) Lymphocytes generated by in vivo priming and in vitro sensitization demonstrate therapeutic efficacy against a murine tumor that lacks apparent immunogenicity. J Immunol 143: 740
19. Yang JC, Perry-Lalley D, Rosenberg SA (1990) An improved method for growing murine tumor-infiltrating lymphocytes with in vivo antitumor activity. J Biol Response Mod 4;9 (2): 149–59
20. Yoshizawa H, Sakai K, Chang AE, Shu S (1991) Activation by anti-CD3 of tumor-draining lymph node cells for specific adoptive immunotherapy. Cell Immunol 134: 473

Cytokines as Possible Adjuvants to Vaccines in Active Specific Immunotherapy for Renal Cell Carcinoma

C.S. McCune[1]

Introduction

Several types of cancer vaccines are being investigated for their use in active specific immunotherapy for cancer patients. These forms of cancer vaccines are listed in Table 1. In renal carcinoma, much of the previous clinical work has been conducted with autologous whole tumor cells [1, 3, 4, 6]. This type of vaccine is prepared by obtaining a sample of the patient's tumor, such as from the nephrectomy specimen, dissociating the tumor cells, radiating them to leave the tumor cells alive but incapable of viable cell division. The underlying concept of why such cancer vaccines may be successfully used in treatment is centered upon the idea of tumor-associated antigens. It is thought that in the transformation from the normal to the malignant cell, there are many genetic changes which occur, such as translocations or point mutations, and as a consequence of these genetic alterations, new molecular products are produced by the cell. It is thought that the molecules expressed on the cell surface undergo changes such that new epitopes are present, and that these epitopes are capable of inducing an immune response directed at these new antigens, called tumor-associated antigens. It is considered that these tumor-associated antigens are usually very weak immunogens, that is, they produce a minimal immune response. Therefore, the growing tumor within the patient has not produced an effective immune response directed at these antigens. The hypothesis is that if these tumor-associated antigens are presented to the immune system in a favorable manner, an effective immune response could be generated. An effective presentation of such a vaccine involves using the skin

[1] University of Rochester Cancer Center, 601 Elmwood Avenue, Box 704, Rochester, NY 14642, USA

G. Staehler S. Pomer (Eds.)
Basic and Clinical Research on Renal Cell Carcinoma

Table 1. Vaccine options for active specific immunotherapy

Whole tumor cell vaccines	
	Autologous tumor cells
	Allogeneic tumor cells
	Allogeneic tumor cells with transfected genes
Subcellular vaccines	
	Lysates of allogeneic tumor cells
	Lysates of virus-infected allogeneic tumor cells
	Tumor antigens, supernatant of allogeneic tumor cultures
	Tumor antigens, biochemically extracted
	Tumor antigens, mirror image anti-idiotype antibodies
	Tumor antigens, gene transfected to vaccinia virus

as an ideal site for acquiring immunity to new antigens, using an adjuvant with the vaccine to facilitate the immune response, and as discussed in the data below, the use of cytokines concurrently with a vaccine may be a way to strengthen the immunologic response. Both interleukin-1 and interleukin-2 (IL-1, IL-2) are T lymphocyte-activating molecules. A postulated mechanism by which these cytokines might work can be summarized as follows: when a cancer vaccine is administered intradermally, it leads to the production of a small number of activated and sensitized T lymphocytes which then circulate and reside in the lymphoid tissues of the body. If one of the lymphocyte-activating molecules such as IL-1 or IL-2 is administered intravenously to the host, this new population of activated lymphocytes can be assisted in its expansion to eventually result in a larger population of sensitized and activated lymphocytes which are directed at the tumor-associated antigens contained in the vaccine. The experimental and clinical studies described below are tests of this general hypothesis.

Interleukin-2 as an Adjuvant to Vaccines in Experimental Studies

Table 2 illustrates an experiment performed by Nunberg [5] in working with a rabies virus vaccine. There is a standardized murine test used for testing these vaccines by the U.S. National Institutes of Health in which the vaccine is administered to the mice at various dilutions, and the mice are subsequently challenged with an intracerebral injection of the rabies virus. The vaccine was administered twice and in one group, IL-2 was given for several days following each

Table 2. Interleukin-2 as an adjuvant to rabies virus vaccine

Vaccine dilution	Rabies Mortality (deaths/group)	
	Vaccine alone	Vaccine plus IL-2 3×10^6 U/kg, BID, IP
undiluted	16/16	0/15
1:5	15/16	5/16
1:25	15/15	13/14
1:125	16/16	16/16

vaccine. When the undiluted vaccine was given, this particular batch was totally ineffective in protecting the mice and 16 out of 16 died from the challenge. In the group that received the IL-2 as a systemic adjuvant with the vaccine, all 15 mice were protected and survived the virus challenge.

Table 3 depicts the experiments performed by Weinberg and associates [7] working with herpes simplex virus vaccines in guinea pigs. The vaccines were administered twice and the IL-2 was administered continuously over a 17-day period, encompassing both vaccine administrations. The guinea pigs were then challenged with the virus in the genital area. There is, again, clear evidence of an improvement in efficacy achieved by the addition of IL-2 to the vaccine regimen.

Table 4 is an experiment which we performed using the line 1 tumor model, a murine spontaneous lung carcinoma. In this study a tumor vaccine consisting of irradiated line 1 tumor cells was administered once followed by subcutaneously administered IL-2 for a period of 10 days. On day 15 the mice were challenged with viable tumor cells and they were observed for the development of tumor nodules at

Table 3. Interleukin-2 as an adjuvant to HSV-2 vaccine in guinea pigs

Antigen Number of doses	Incidence of infection	
	Vaccine plus rIL-2 5×10^4 U, s.c., daily $\times$ 17 days	Vaccine alone
control	8/10	9/10
RGD $\times$ 2	4/10	10/10
RGD $\times$ 3	1/8	5/8
HSV $\times$ 2	2/10	8/10
HSV $\times$ 3	0/8	6/8

Table 4. IL-2 given for 10 days following the vaccine

Group	Vaccine	IL-2[a]	Mean survival (Days ± SE)[b]	Tumor free/ Total (0/0)[b]
1	–	–	11.10 ± 0.65	0/10 (0)
2	3×10^5 TC	–	11.80 ± 1.30	0/10 (0)
3	3×10^5 TC	300 U dl-10	20.20 ± 3.58[c]	2/10 (20)
4	3×10^5 TC	1000 U dl-10	22.20 ± 4.04[c]	3/10 (30)[d]
5	3×10^5 TC	4000 U dl-10	24.80 ± 3.68[c]	3/10 (30)[d]

[a] Given i.c. distant from vaccine.
[b] Statistical comparisons with group 2 are given.
[c] $p < 0.05$, [d] $p = 0.02$.

the challenge sites for up to 40 days. By prior experience we know that no tumors appear in control animals after approximately 30 days. There was a significant delay in tumor appearance and a portion of the animals were rendered tumor free. At doses of IL-2 going ten fold higher, we could not improve upon this result.

Interleukin-2 as an Adjuvant to Vaccines for Renal Cell Carcinoma

IL-2 was the first cytokine to become available for clinical studies and we are currently underway with a protocol for renal cell carcinoma and melanoma based on these interesting preclinical experiments. An outline of this clinical study is shown in Fig. 1. The dose of cyclophosphamide is $100\,mg/m^2$ and it is given for its potential suppressor function inhibition. The vaccine contains 10^7 autologous irradiated tumor cells with the adjuvant Ovamid provided by Ribi ImmunoChem Inc. (Hamilton, MT, USA) The IL-2 is administered intra-

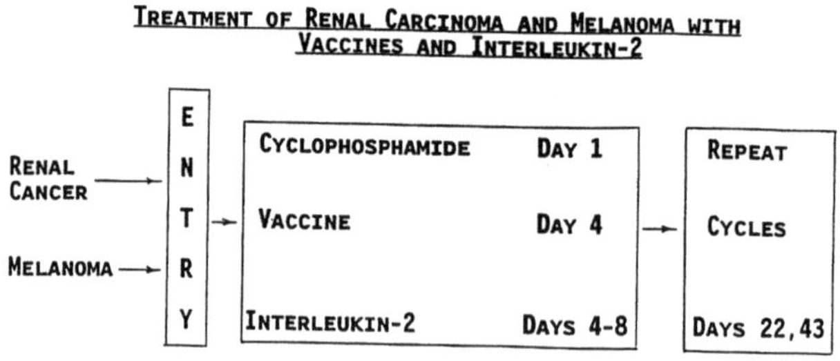

Fig. 1. Outline of the clinical protocol

Table 5. Vaccine and IL-2 protocol

Dose of IL-2	Responses/ # Patients	Type of Response
6×10^5 IU/m^2/day	0/3	
18×10^5 IU/m^2/day	2/4	MR melanoma: 1 lung CR, 1 skin PR, 1 axilla P MR renal: 1 lung CR, 1 adrenal P
6×10^6 IU/m^2/day	1/5	MR melanoma: 2 skin CR, 2 skin PR, 1 skin NC, 2 skin P
18×10^6 IU/m^2/day	2/2	PR renal: 7 lung CR, 3 lung PR PR renal: 4 lung CR, 1 lung PR, 1 adrenal NC

CR, complete response; MR, mixed response; NC, no change;
PR, partial response; P, progression

venously as a continuous infusion for a 5-day period following each vaccine. Table 5 shows the results in this study for the first 14 patients which have entered. Three interesting mixed responses were seen at the lower doses of IL-2 in which some lesions regressed, while others did not, an occurrence similar to what we have seen in previous vaccine studies [3]. The response seen in a renal carcinoma patient at the second dose level was followed by resection of an unresponsive adrenal metastasis and this patient has had no progression of disease for over 12 months. Our experience with the highest dose of IL-2 is just beginning, but is proving to be very interesting. The first two patients which have completed this treatment have both had excellent responses. The response of the first patient is illustrated in Fig. 2. Ten measurable lesions were selected to follow from the pretreatment CT scan of his chest. After two treatments with the vaccine and IL-2, all lesions were distinctly smaller and after three treatments, 7 of the 10 lung metastases had completely regressed. The radiologist read this last CT scan of the chest as being totally clear of any metastases, however, by serially following where we knew they had been, we felt that some traces remained, as has been indicated by the figure. The second patient has also had an excellent response with 4 out of 5 lung lesions completely regressing after only two treatments. The responses in both of these patients were very rapid. In past experience with vaccines, we have often seen the regressions continuing for several months, so they may improve still further. A logical question to ask is whether these responses could be due to the IL-2 alone or the vaccine

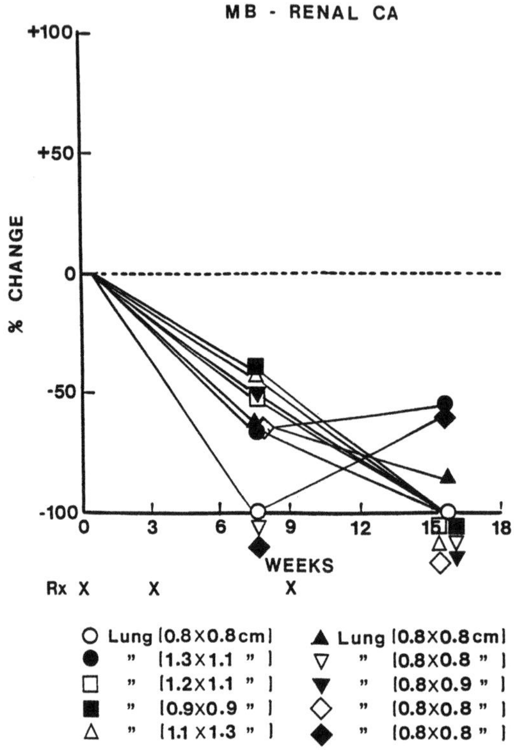

Fig. 2. Regression of 10 metastatic lung lesions. The initial measurement is given with the symbol for each lesion

alone. Our highest dose of IL-2 is approximately 25% of the dose used by the Rosenberg group at Bethesda for patients treated with IL-2 alone, and with that dose they did achieve a 22% response rate. Our two previous studies with vaccine alone achieved a 23% response rate overall. Therefore, only as our experience with the current protocol enlarges will we be able to determine whether a higher response rate is being achieved.

Interleukin-1 as an Adjuvant to Vaccines in an Experimental Model

IL-1 is also thought to be one of the key molecules involved in T-lymphocyte activation. We have tested the use of this cytokine in our line 1 murine model [2]. The experiment shown in Table 6 was

Table 6. IL-1α given for 1, 3 or 8 days, and comparison of administration at the vaccine site or a distant site

Group	Vaccine	IL-1α	Site[a]	Mean Survival (Days ± S.E.)[b]	Tumor Free/ Total (%)[b]
1	–	–	–	12.70 ± 0.423	0/10 (0)
2	3×10^5 TC	–	–	17.80 ± 2.76	1/10 (10)
3	3×10^5 TC	360 ng d1	vaccine	22.19 ± 4.52	2/9 (22)
4	3×10^5 TC	360 ng d1,3,5	vaccine	26.90 ± 3.82	4/10 (40)
5	3×10^5 TC	360 ng d1-8	vaccine	31.00 ± 4.07[c]	6/10 (60)[d]
6	3×10^5 TC	720 ng d1,3,5	vaccine	21.20 ± 2.50	1/10 (10)
7	3×10^5 TC	360 ng d1,3,5	distant	30.33 ± 4.30[e]	5/9 (56)[f]

[a] IL-1α was administered either at the vaccine site or on the leg.
[b] Statistical comparisons with group 2 are indicated.
[c] $p < 0.02$, [d] $p = 0.02$, [e] $p < 0.05$, [f] $p = 0.03$.

conducted by giving the vaccine on day 1, the IL-1 on subsequent days as indicated. The site of administration of the IL-1 was either at the vaccine site on the chest wall or at a distant location on the leg. We had originally thought that the IL-1 should be administered daily at the vaccine site. However, in this experiment, as seen in group 7, administration of IL-1 on the leg was equally effective with group 4, in which the same dose and schedule were used but the IL-1 was administered at the vaccine site. Also in this experiment, of note is group 6 in which we went to our highest dose of IL-1. These mice were quite ill and as seen, the adjuvant effect was lost at this very high dose.

Table 7 is an experiment in which both IL-1α and IL-1β were used and the effect of these cytokines alone was compared with their use in

Table 7. IL-1α and IL-1β given alone or with vaccines

Group	Vaccine	IL-1α (ng)	IL-1β (ng)	Mean Survival (Days ± S.E.)[a]	Tumor Free/ Total (%)[a]
1	–	–	–	13.11 ± 0.992	0/9 (0)
2	3×10^5 TC	–	–	17.10 ± 2.848	1/10 (10)
3	–	360 d1-8	–	13.10 ± 0.547	0/10 (0)
4	–	–	360 d1-8	14.60 ± 0.763	0/10 (0)
5	3×10^5 TC	360 d1-8	–	25.50 ± 4.146[bf]	4/10 (40)[c]
6	3×10^5 TC	–	360 d1-8	35.80 ± 3.757[d]	8/10 (80)[e]

[a] Statistical comparisons with group 2 are indicated.
[b] $p < 0.2$, [c] $p = 0.12$, [d] $p < 0.001$, [e] $p = 0.002$,
[f] $p < 0.05$ compared with group 3.

combination with the vaccine. Again, the tumor challenge was given on day 15, which is 7 days after the last doses of IL-1. We see that the cytokines alone produced no effect on survival, but both types of IL-1 were effective when used as systemic adjuvants in conjunction with the vaccines. The doses of both types of IL-1 were based on weight rather than specific activity and this result does not serve as evidence that one type of IL-1 is superior to the other.

One concern in using IL-1 is that when administered systemically, it can produce toxic side effects at the higher dose levels. We weighed animals in each group in the experiment shown in Table 7 and found that at the 360-ng dose, both IL-1α and IL-1β did prevent the animals from eating and acquiring their normal weight gain.

An additional question addressed in the animal studies was what time period following the administration of a vaccine is best suited for the administration of IL-1. In Table 8, the results of an experiment are shown in which IL-1 was administered following the vaccine on day 1. The IL-1 was given at three different time periods as indicated in Table 8. We noted that administering IL-1 on days 1–5 or days 6–10 produced an adjuvant effect and improved the efficacy of the vaccine. Delaying administration of IL-1 to begin on day 11 and continue through day 15 did not contribute to vaccine efficacy. This suggests that IL-1's most useful role is during the initial response to antigens when the lymphocytes are becoming activated and expanded following stimulation by administration of the antigen.

Table 9 shows the results of an experiment in which two additional questions were addressed. The first question was whether a fragment of the IL-1 molecule could be used in place of the whole molecule. This would be desirable for the purpose of retaining the immunologic effect but avoiding toxic side effects. As seen, the fragment 163–171 was effective at high doses but unfortunately, did also produce side

Table 8. IL-1α given at three time periods following the vaccines

Group	Vaccine	IL-1α	Mean survival (Days ± S.E.)[a]	Tumor Free/ Total (%)[a]
1	–	–	11.22 ± 0.434	0/9 (0)
2	3×10^5 TC	–	13.60 ± 0.702	0/10 (0)
3	3×10^5 TC	360 ng d1-5	26.70 ± 4.730[b]	5/10 (50)[b]
4	3×10^5 TC	360 ng d6-10	23.90 ± 3.766[c]	3/10 (30)[d]
5	3×10^5 TC	360 ng d11-15	15.70 ± 1.096	0/10 (0)

[a] Statistical comparisons with group 2 are indicated.
[b] $p < 0.01$, [c] $p < 0.02$, [d] $p = 0.06$.

Table 9. The adjuvant effect of IL-1β or the peptide fragment 163-171

Group	Vaccine	Peptide of IL-1β (ng)	IL-1β(ng)	Mean Survival (Days ± S.E.)[a]	Tumor Free/ Total (%)[a]	% Weight Change
1	–	–	–	14.90 ± 1.02	0/10 (0)	+6
2	3×10^5 TC	–	–	17.00 ± 0.97	0/10 (0)	+5
3	3×10^5 TC	360 d1-8	–	17.00 ± 0.68	0/10 (0)	+5
4	3×10^5 TC	3600 d1-8	–	24.90 ± 3.50[b]	3/10 (30)	+4
5	3×10^5 TC	36000 d1-8	–	22.60 ± 3.01	2/10 (20)	+3
6	3×10^5 TC	100000 d1-8	–	29.80 ± 3.69[c]	5/10 (50)[c]	+1
7	3×10^5 TC	–	120 d1-8	33.80 ± 3.66[d]	7/10 (70)[e]	+6
8	3×10^5 TC	–	360 d1-8	40.00 ± 0.00[d]	10/10 (100)[f]	+0.6

[a] Statistical comparisons with group 2 are indicated.
[b] $p < 0.05$, [c] $p < 0.01$, [d] $p < 0.001$
[e] $p = 0.001$, [f] $p < 0.0004$.

effects such that the animals did not gain weight compared with control animals. In groups 7 and 8 two doses of IL-1 were compared. We see that at the 120-ng dose a strong adjuvant effect was obtained, such that 70% of the animals became tumor free and at this lower dose, there was no impairment of weight gain. This indicates that a dose was found which was well tolerated and yet could greatly facilitate the effectiveness of the tumor cell vaccine.

Summary

The preclinical studies described above indicate that lymphocyte-activating cytokines such as IL-1 and IL-2 may represent effective ways to improve the immune response to poorly immunogenic vaccines. Excessively toxic doses might prove to be detrimental and abrogate the beneficial effects of the adjuvant role. In the murine model the first 10 days following the vaccine is a critical period of time in which the adjuvant IL-1 function can be achieved. The phase I study of this concept as applied to metastatic renal carcinoma is under way and showing some interesting results at this early point. An expansion of this study and subsequent comparative studies to determine the contribution of IL-2 versus vaccine versus the combination will be necessary to determine if this concept can be usefully applied in the treatment of human diseases such as cancer.

Acknowledgements. This work is supported in part by a USPHS Grant RR-00044, General Clinical Research Centers Branch, NIH, and by a gift from the Glen and Maude Wyman Potter Foundation.

References

1. Adler A, Gillon G, Lurie H et al. (1987) Active specific immunotherapy of renal cell carcinoma patients: a prospective randomized study of hormono-immuno versus hormonotherapy. Preliminary report of immunological and clinical aspects. J Biol Response Mod 6: 610–624
2. McCune CS, Marquis DM (1990) Interleukin 1 as an adjuvant for active specific immunotherapy in a murine tumor model. Cancer 50: 1212–1215
3. McCune CS, Schapira DV, Henshaw EC (1981) Specific immunotherapy of advanced renal carcinoma: evidence for the polyclonality of metastases. Cancer 47: 1984–1987

4. McCune C, O'Donnell R, Marquis D, Sahasrabudhe D (1990) Renal cell carcinoma treated by vaccines for active specific immunotherapy: correlation of survival with skin testing by autologous tumor cells. Cancer Immunol Immunother 32: 562–566
5. Nunberg JH, Doyle MV, Newell AD, Anderson GA, York CJ (1988) Interleukin-2 as an adjuvant to vaccination. J Cell Biochem (Suppl) 12B: 12
6. Scharfe T, Muller S, Riedmiller H, Jacobi GH, Hohenfellner R (1989) Immunotherapy of metastasizing renal cell carcinoma. Urol Int 44: 1–4
7. Weinberg A, Merigan TC (1988) Recombinant interleukin 2 as an adjuvant for vaccine-induced protection. J Immunol 140: 294–299

Tumor Infiltrating Lymphocytes in Renal Cell Cancer

G.P. Haas[1], J.E. Pontes[1], and A. Belldegrun[2]

Introduction

For the past decade the immunotherapy approach to the treatment of solid cancers resistant to conventional treatment modalities has proven to be of benefit, particularly in melanoma and metastatic renal cell cancer. Cancer patients were treated with the lymphokine interleukin-2 (IL-2) alone, or in combination with other lymphokines in order to activate the patient's immune system against the cancer. Alternatively, autologous circulating lymphocytes obtained by leukapheresis of the patient were activated and expanded with IL-2 in vitro, leading to the generation of lymphokine-activated killer (LAK) cells. These LAK cells capable of mediating a high degree of antitumor activity were reinfused to the patients in combination with IL-2 administration, thus providing the patient with a large pool of killer cells. Following LAK cell therapy for renal cell cancer 35% partial and complete response rates have been achieved with many durable responses and several patients who are still in remission after 3 years [21].

It has been noted that most solid tumors, including renal cell cancer, are associated with variable degrees of lymphocytic infiltrates [27]. Based on the assumption that the infiltrating lymphocytes may have a role in antitumor activity, intensive efforts have been initiated to isolate, characterize and expand this cell population. Tumor infiltrating lymphocytes (TIL) are predominantly T cells that can be

[1] Section of Urological Oncology, Department of Urology, Wayne State University, School of Medicine, Detroit, MI 48201, USA
[2] Cancer Immunotherapy Program School of Medicine, Jonsson Comprehensive Cancer Center 10833 Le Compte Avenue, Los Angeles, CA 90024-1738, USA

G. Staehler S. Pomer (Eds.)
Basic and Clinical Research on Renal Cell Carcinoma

isolated from solid tumors when single cell suspensions are cultured in the presence of IL-2 [13, 17, 28]. Unlike LAK cells, TIL can be expanded in large numbers and maintained in long term cultures. Moreover, TIL were demonstrated to be up to a 100 times more effective in their therapeutic potency than LAK cells on a cell to cell basis [19, 23]. TIL mediate cytotoxic activity against autologous and allogeneic tumor targets in vitro. TIL isolated from melanomas often demonstrate specific, MHC-restricted cytotoxicity in 4-h chromium release assays [14, 17, 22, 26]; however, most renal cell carcinoma derived TIL kill in a non-MHC-restricted manner [3]. In animal models, the efficiency of TIL therapy required pretreatment of the host with either sublethal total body irradiation or the immunosuppressive chemotherapeutic agent cyclophosphamide [19, 23]. The rationale for the pretreatment is still unclear and may include the elimination of host suppressor cells [18], reduction in the tumor burden by direct or other antitumor effect [7], or the creation of increased lymphoid space to allow for the adoptive transfer of large quantity of cells. Adoptively transferred TIL have been shown to have long-term survival in mice [1] and are found to preferentially localize to metastases in melanoma patients [10, 11]. In clinical trials involving 20 patients with metastatic melanoma, Rosenberg observed one complete response of greater than 13 months in duration and 10 partial responses of 2–9 months in duration [20]. These promising results formed the basis for the efforts to develop TIL therapy for metastatic renal cell cancer.

TIL Culture Techniques

The initiation of TIL culture requires the procurement of fresh tumor tissue. TIL can be grown from both primary and metastatic lesions. To minimize tissue ischemia during nephrectomy, the vascular pedicle is divided after the kidney is completely mobilized. While this technique may seem contrary to the standard surgical approach for a cancer operation, it should be kept in mind that these patients already have systemic metastases at the time of the surgery. The resected tumor specimen is kept sterile and transferred to the laboratory where it is processed in a sterile laminar flow hood. After sufficient tissue is submitted for histological confirmation, the tumor is dissected free of the surrounding normal parenchyma, minced with sterile instruments into pieces of less than 1 cm^3 in size and digested overnight in an enzyme solution containing collagenase, hyaluronidase and DNAse.

The cells are washed, and viable tumor and mononuclear cells are separated by Ficoll-Hypaque density gradient centrifugation. The cells are incubated at a concentration of 2.5 to 5 × 10^5 cells/ml in the presence of IL-2 for TIL expansion. After 10–14 days of culture, a pure population of lymphoid cells devoid of tumor cells are present. The goal of these cultures is to expand the TIL population to 10^{10} to 10^{12} cells, which is the number generally used for adoptive transfer.

TIL can be grown in a variety of basic media. Initial studies utilized RPMI 1640 with 10% human serum, but consequently the addition of 20% conditioned medium (supernatant of LAK cells cultured from normal donors) was found to increase both the percentage of successful cultures and the total cell expansion (Fig. 1) [12, 25]. Growth variations attributed to the use of different batches of human serum and the concern over the potential risk of the transmission of infectious agents led to the development of serum-free medium for TIL expansion [16]. TIL expand very well in commercially available serum-free media; however, slight variations in cell populations and their in vitro activity have been noted [12]. These changes do not occur with sufficient consistency to allow selection of desired phenotypes by choice of the medium. Thus, most TIL cultures intended for therapy are currently expanded in serum-free medium.

TIL grown for therapy have been traditionally cultured in gas permeable bags in a CO_2 incubator at 37 °C. The cultures are fed periodically as the cells increase in density and the color of the pH indicator changes. The cells are split into larger bags by diluting the old medium with fresh medium containing the desired amount of IL-2 and other factors. Expansion takes 4–6 weeks, and it is evident that very large volumes of medium, numerous bags and space are required to grow TIL under these cumbersome conditions.

More recently, the new technology of hollow fiber bioreactors became available to grow cells in large numbers with continuously circulating medium. This is a very compact, entirely closed system in which the medium can be completely replaced once it is utilized. This system is capable of expanding the necessary number of cells in the required period of time and is a major advance in terms of space, supplies, manpower, and sterility.

Phenotype of TIL Cultures

There are several methods available to assess the phenotype of the initial cell population present in the tumor specimen prior to TIL a

b

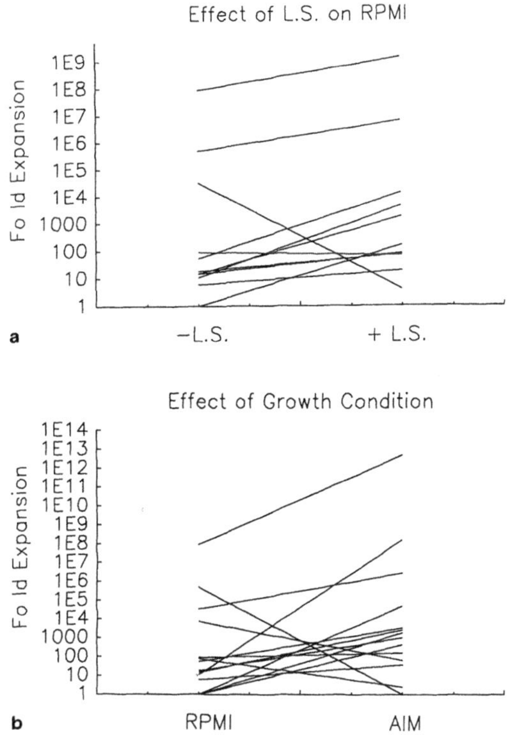

Fig. 1a, b. Expansion of TIL grown under various culture conditions. Each *line* represents expansion of TIL derived from a different patient. **a** RPMI with 10% human serum vs. RPMI, 10% human serum and 20% supernatant from 3-day LAK cell cultures from healthy donors. – L.S., without LAK supernatant, + L.S. with LAK supernatant. **b** RPMI with 10% human serum vs. AIM V (Gibco)

expansion. These methods utilize commercially available antibodies directed against cell surface antigens. Immunohisto-chemical analysis of permanent histological sections allows the assessment of the original cell population present immediately adjacent to tumor areas processed for the TIL culture. The cellular components of the single cell suspension obtained after enzymatic digestion and density gradient separation can be determined and phenotyped using techniques of immunocytochemistry or flow cytometry.

During the first week of culture in IL-2 the cell composition undergoes major shifts. Tumor cells, B cells and macrophages disappear from the culture medium, while lymphocytes become the major component of the culture. The CD3-/CD56^{+} NK cells are markedly reduced in most TIL cultures and the culture consists almost exclusively of $CD3^+$ T cells. The ratio of $CD4^+$ to $CD8^+$ cells is variable, and while $CD8^+$ cells often predominate in melanoma TIL, a majority of $CD4^+$ T cells are present in renal cell cancer TILs expanded in high-dose IL-2. Some cultures contain a significant fraction of $CD3^+/CD56^+$ T-cell subpopulation that mediates MHC-unrestricted, LAK-like cytotoxic activity [9]. In most cultures, the majority of cells are $HLA\text{-}DR^+$ up to 40–60 days but this population decreases with longer term incubation. IL-2 receptor levels vary, but also tend to decline in aging cultures [3].

In order to better determine the function of certain cell populations in the immune response, and to select for those TIL which may have more potent activity, different methods have been devised to enrich TIL cultures in one or another cell subpopulation. Animal studies demonstrated that cytotoxic lymphocytes are more likely to grow out in cultures stimulated by low-dose IL-2 (<50 U/ml) [2]. Unfortunately, TIL expansion in low-dose IL-2 is very poor and rarely sufficient to yield the necessary cell numbers for adoptive transfer. Whiteside described TIL grown in low-dose IL-2 in the presence of tumor necrosis factor (TNF), and this lymphokine combination resulted in selective outgrowth of CD8+ cells [15].

The lymphokine IL-4 can also augment the expansion of TIL grown in low-dose IL-2. Studies conducted at UCLA demonstrated a significant increase in lymphocyte proliferation in the presence of IL-4 (Belldegrun et al., manuscript submitted for publication). IL-4 increased the expansion of cultures receiving low-dose (20 U/ml) of IL-2 (average increase of 6.5-fold expansion, $p < 0.01$), but did not further increase the proliferation of high-dose (1000 U/ml) cultures. Combination of low-dose IL-2 and IL-4 (200 U/ml) promoted lymphocyte growth significantly better than high-dose IL-2 alone. TIL grown in the presence of IL-4 significantly reduced the level of nonspecific, non-MHC-restricted antitumor activity, while it did not affect the level of autologous killing (Fig. 2). The greatest total-fold expansion was seen in those cultures containing the combination of IL-4, low-dose IL-2 and irradiated autologous tumor cells, which exhibited a 5.22 ± 2.44 greater-fold expansion than TIL irradiated in the standard 1000 U/ml of IL-2 alone. These results suggest that IL-4 and irradiated autologous tumor cells are effective growth simulators, when used in combination with a low-dose IL-2 regimen, and may be of significant benefit for growing activated TIL from patients with renal cell carcinoma.

Alternatively, T-cell subpopulations can be isolated from TIL

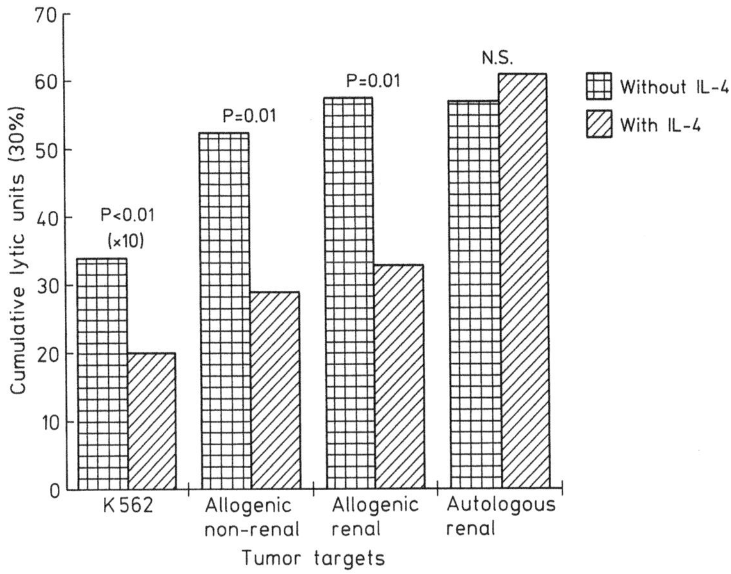

Fig. 2. Effect of IL-4 on cytotoxicity by TIL. IL-4 reduces non-specific antitumor activity against allogeneic targets while it does not affect the level of autologous killing

cultures and expanded selectively. Finke et al., described the technique of positive selection for $CD3^+/CD4^+$ or $CD3^+/CD8^+$ T cells by adherence to antibody-coated beads [9]. Pure populations separated at the initiation of the cultures, expanded well in IL-2 and maintained their phenotype as well as their cytolytic activities upon further culture. Wong et al., utilized bispecific antibodies (anti-CD3: anti-CD4) to cause selective cytolysis of $CD4^+$ cells while concurrently expanding and activating the residual $CD8^+$ cells, or conversely, anti-CD3: anti-CD8 antibody to cause cytolysis of $CD8^+$ cells and select for the $CD4^+$ subpopulation. The final populations were 86%–97% pure $CD3^+/CD4^+$ or $CD3^+/CD8^+$ T cells which retained their ability to expand and to lyse tumor target cells in chromium release assays [29].

TIL Antitumor Lytic Ability

The gold standard of assessing in vitro cytotoxicity has been the 4-h chromium release assay. Unlike melanoma TIL, which frequently demonstrate specific, MHC-restricted cytotoxicity for the autologous tumor target, TIL from renal cell cancer are usually just as effective against a variety of allogeneic fresh or cultured tumor targets as against the autologous tumor. That some renal tumors harbor specific TIL has been demonstrated by Belldegrun, who thoroughly characterized a specific clone [5]. The most likely explanation for this phenomenon may be that TIL clones specific for the autologous tumor cell are present at very low frequencies in renal cell cancer and are difficult to detect at the bulk culture level.

Cytolytic activity is usually expressed as lytic units/10^6 cells. One lytic unit is defined as the number of effector cells required to produce a certain degree of lysis of the target cell population. The degree of lysis selected varies from author to author and is usually in the range of 15%–30%.

Exclusive reliance on the 4-h chromium release assay to measure cytotoxicity has been recently questioned. Finke described a series of experiments where TIL studied in a 4-h chromium release assay failed to demonstrate any cytotoxic activity; however, when the assay was carried out for 18 h, or the cells were tested in a 3-day coincubation assay with target cells, they were found to be highly cytotoxic [9]. While the most potent cytotoxic cells were of the $CD3^-/CD56^+$ NK-cell or $CD3^+/CD56^+$ T-cell phenotypes, cytotoxic activity was also mediated by the $CD3^+/CD56^-$ T-cell populations. Both the $CD3^+/CD4^+/CD8^-$ and $CD3^+/CD4^-/CD8^+$ T cells demonstrated comparable lytic activity.

Cytolytic activity of TIL may also be enhanced by modifications of the target cells. Stotter demonstrated that TIL activity can be greatly increased by pretreatment of the target cells with TNF and interferons (Fig. 3) [24]. Presumably this type of pretreatment could result in upregulation of certain tumor antigens or MHC antigens which may allow for improved recognition and cytotoxicity by the TIL. The clinical implications of this hypothesis are currently being tested in human trials using TNF and interferons in combination with TIL.

Repeated stimulation of the TIL culture by irradiated autologous tumor has been attempted to increase TIL specificity [9]. Belldegrun has recently examined the growth and cytolytic patterns of bulk culture TIL from human renal cell carcinoma cultured side by side in either low (20 U/ml) or high (1000 U/ml) dose IL-2, with or without irradiated autologous tumor stimulation. By 55 days in culture, TIL grown in the presence of IL-2 without tumor stimulation lost their lytic activity, whereas those exposed to tumor stimulation maintained high levels of cytotoxicity against autologous and/or allogeneic tumor

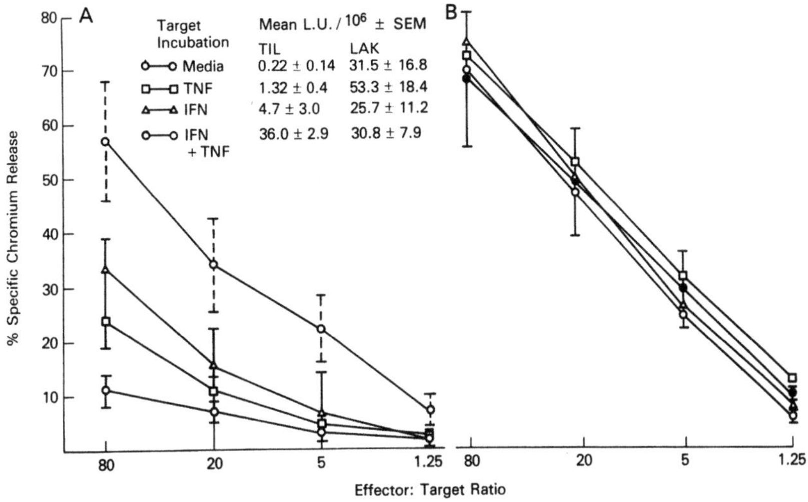

Fig. 3. Pretreatment of target cells by TNF and IFN enhances cytotoxicity by TIL but not LAK cells. (Adopted from Stotter et al. [24])

targets. Only TIL grown with low-dose IL-2 and autologous tumor maintained long-term specific cytotoxicity against the autologous tumor, even upon cryopreservation and regrowth (Fig. 4; Belldegrun et al., manuscript submitted for publication). Thus, an antigen-specific cytotoxicity against the autologous tumor does in fact exist within the renal cell cancer tumors. Innovative approaches to expand and improve potency of these cells could result in increased efficacy of adoptive cancer immunotherapy.

The major pitfall in assessing TIL characteristics by phenotypic analysis or cytotoxicity assays is that none of the currently available studies correlate directly with in vivo activity. Despite intensive research into the characteristics of the patient, the tumor, and the TIL generated from this tumor we cannot yet predict which patients are likely to respond. Recent evidence suggests, however, that profiles of lymphokine secretion may provide a useful marker for functionally characterizing different T-cell subsets and may provide correlates of the in vivo antitumor effects of these cells when TIL are adoptively transferred into cancer-bearing patients [4].

Phase I trials of TIL therapy of renal cell cancer have been initiated at several institutions including the National Cancer Institute, the Cleveland Clinic Foundation, the M.D. Anderson Cancer Center, and UCLA. Most of the toxicity encountered is related to IL-2 infusion.

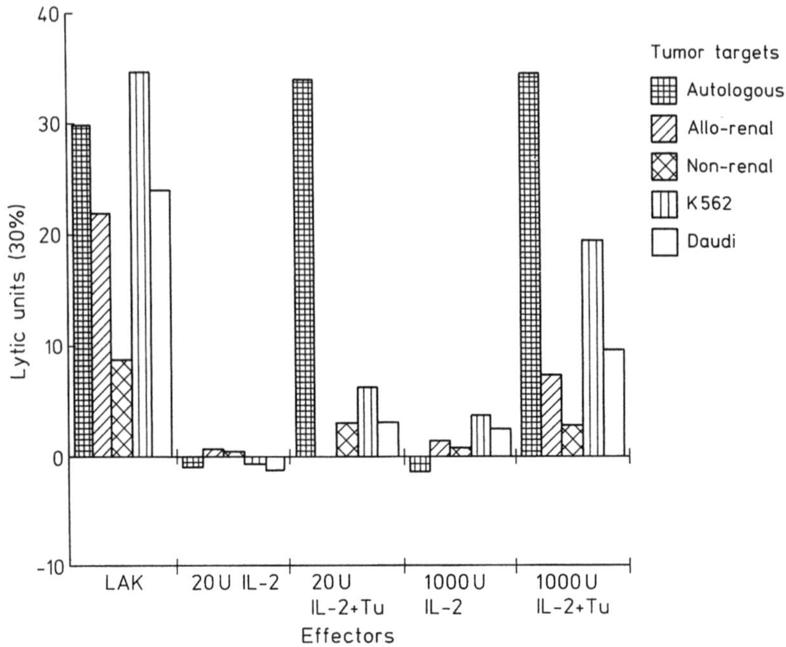

Fig. 4. Cytolytic activity of TIL grown under four different culture conditions and tested on day 55 in culture against a variety of tumor targets. LAK effectors serve as a positive control. Addition of irradiated autologous tumor maintains specific cytotoxicity

Fever and chills are the only side effects associated with TIL administration and these are easily controlled with meperidine. There have not been any treatment-related deaths reported.

Among 18 patients evaluated for clinical response at the Cleveland Clinic Foundation, only a minor response was seen [6]. In each case, more than 10^9 cells were infused. The cells were derived from primary or metastatic disease and had similar ability to expand. The large majority of cells exhibited $CD3^+$ phenotype. The percentage of cells exhibiting $CD4^+$ and $CD8^+$ phenotype varied significantly from one patient to another [8]. Only a few patients had TILs consisting of NK cells. The cytolytic activity of the cultured TILs were evaluated against autologous tumor and allogeneic cell lines. The majority of cultures demonstrated non-MHC-restricted lytic activity. In one case, cytotoxicity was specific for the autologous tumor cells.

Efforts at UCLA are now under way to improve the potency of TIL immunotherapy by in vivo lymphokine priming prior to nephrectomy and to infuse these primed TIL in combination with IL-2 and interferon-alpha.

The preliminary data so far have demonstrated the feasibility and safety of administering TIL to patients with renal cell carcinoma. Further efforts to improve the expansion of desired cell subpopulations will lead to increased efficacy. It is the hope that the preliminary studies discussed in this chapter will form the basis of adoptive immunotherapy for the treatment of patients with advanced renal cell cancer.

References

1. Alexander RB, Rosenberg SA (1990) Long term survival of adoptively transferred tumor-infiltrating lymphocytes in mice. J Immunol 145: 1615–1620
2. Barth RJ, Bock SN, Mule JJ, Rosenberg SA (1990) Unique murine tumor associated antigens identified by tumor infiltrating lymphocytes. J Immunol 144: 1531
3. Belldegrun A, Muul LM, Rosenberg SA (1988) Interleukin 2 expanded tumor-infiltrating lymphocytes in human renal cell cancer: isolation, characterization, and antitumor activity. Cancer Res 48: 206–214
4. Belldegrun A, Kasid A, Uppenkamp M, Topalian SL, Rosenberg SA (1989) Human tumor infiltrating lymphocytes: analysis of lymphokine mRNA expression and relevance to cancer immunotherapy. J Immunol 142: 4520–4526
5. Belldegrun A, Uppenkamp A, Rosenberg SA (1990) Lymphokine mRNA profile and functional analysis of a human CD4+ clone with unique antitumor specificity isolated from renal cell carcinoma ascitic fluid. Cancer Immunol Immunother 31 (1): 1–10
6. Bukowski RM, Murthy S, Rayman P, et al. (1991) Clinical results and characterization of tumor infiltrating lymphocytes with or without recombinant interleukin-2 in human metastatic renal cell carcinoma. Cancer Res 51: 4199–4205.
7. Cameron RB, Spiess PJ, Rosenberg SA (1990) Synergistic antitumor activity of tumor infiltrating lymphocytes, interleukin-2, and local tumor irradiation: studies on the mechanism of action. J Exp Med 171: 249–263
8. Finke JH, Tubbs R, Connelly R, Pontes E, Montie J (1988) Tumor infiltrating lymphocytes in patients with renal cell carcinoma. In: Battisto J, Plate J, Shearer G (eds) Cytotoxic T cells: biology and relevance to disease. New York Academy of Science pp 387–394
9. Finke JH, Rayman P, Alexander J, et al. (1990) Characterization of the cytolytic activity of CD4+ and CD8+ tumor-infiltrating lymphocytes in human renal cell carcinoma. Cancer Res 50: 2363–2370
10. Fisher B, Packard BS, Read EF, et al. (1989) Tumor localization of adoptively transferred indium-111 labeled tumor infiltrating lymphocytes in patients with metastatic melanoma. J Clin Oncol 7: 250–261

11. Griffith KD, Read EJ, Carrasquillo JA, et al. (1989) In vivo distribution of adoptively transferred indium-111-labeled tumor infiltrating lymphocytes in patients with metastatic melanoma. JNCI 81: 1709–1717
12. Haas GP, Solomon D, Rosenberg SA (1990) Tumor-infiltrating lymphocytes from nonrenal urological malignancies. Cancer Immunol Immunother 30: 342–350
13. Itoh K, Tilden AB, Balch CM (1986) Interleukin 2 activation of cytotoxic T-lymphocytes infiltrating into human metastatic melanomas. Cancer Res 46: 3011–3017
14. Itoh K, Platsoucas CD, Balch CM (1988) Autologous tumor-specific cytotoxic T lymphocytes in the infiltrate of human metastatic melanomas. Activation by interleukin 2 and autologous tumor cells and involvement of the T cell receptor. J Exp Med 168: 1419–1441
15. Li WY, Lusheng S, Kanbour A, Herberman RB, Whiteside TL (1989) Lymphocytes infiltrating human ovarian tumors: synergy between tumor necrosis factor and interleukin 2 in the generation of CD8+ effectors from tumor-infiltrating lymphocytes. Cancer Res 49: 5979–5985
16. Muul LL, Nason-Burchenal K, Hyatt C, Schwarz S, Slavin D, Director EP, Rosenberg SA (1987) Studies of serum-free culture medium in the generation of lymphokine activated killer cells J Immunol Methods 105: 183–192
17. Muul LM, Spiess PJ, Director EP, Rosenberg SA (1987) Identification of specific cytolytic immune response against autologous tumor in humans bearing malignant melanoma J Immunol 138: 989–995
18. North RJ (1984) Gamma-irradiation facilitates the expression of adoptive immunotherapy of an established tumor by eliminating suppressor T cells. Cancer Immunol Immunother 16: 175–181
19. Rosenberg SA, Spiess P, Lafreniere R (1986) A new approach to the adoptive immunotherapy of cancer with infiltrating lymphocytes. Science 233: 1318–1321
20. Rosenberg SA, Packard BS, Aebersold PM, et al. (1988) Use of tumor-infiltrating lymphocytes and interleukin-2 in the immunotherapy of patients with metastatic melanoma. N Engl J Med 319: 1676–1680
21. Rosenberg SA, Lotze MT, Yang JC, Aebersold PM, Linehan WM, Seipp CA, White DE (1989) Experience with the use of high-dose interleukin-2 in the treatment of 652 cancer patients. Ann Surg 210: 474–485
22. Slingluff CL, Darrow TL, Seigler HF (1987) Human T cells specifically activated against autologous malignant melanoma. Arch Surg 122: 1207–1411
23. Spiess PJ, Yang JC, Rosenberg SA (1987) In vivo antitumor activity of tumor infiltrating lymphocytes expanded in recombinant interleukin 2. JNCI 75: 1067–1075
24. Stotter H, Wiebke EA, Tomita S, Belldegrun A, Topalian S, Rosenberg SA, Lotze MT (1989) Cytokines alter target cell susceptibility to lysis. II. Evaluation of tumor infiltrating lymphocytes. J Immunol 142: 1767–1773
25. Topalian SL, Muul LM, Solomon D, Rosenberg SA (1987) Expansion of human tumor infiltrating lymphocytes for use in immunotherapy trials. J Immunol Methods 102: 127–141

26. Topalian SL, Solomon D, Rosenberg SA (1989) Tumor-specific cytolysis by lymphocytes infiltrating human melanoma. J Immunol 142: 3714–3725
27. Vose BM, Moore M (1985) Human tumor-infiltrating lymphocytes: a marker of host response. Semin Hematol 11: 27–40
28. Whiteside TL, Miescher S, Hurlimann J, Moretta L, Fliedner V von (1986) Separation, phenotyping and limiting dilution analysis of T-lymphocytes infiltrating human solid tumors. Int J Cancer 37: 803–811
29. Wong JT, Pinto CE, Gifford JD, Kurnick JT, Kradin RL (1989) Characterization of the CD4+ and CD8+ tumor infiltrating lymphocytes propagated with bispecific monoclonal antibodies. J Immunol 143: 3404–3411

Combined Vaccination with Autologous Tumor Material and Subcutaneously Administered rIL-2 and rIFN-α-2b in the Treatment of Renal Cell Carcinoma

S. Pomer[1], R. Thiele[1], G. Riedasch[1], M. Wiesel[1], V. Schirrmacher[2], and G. Staehler[1]

Introduction

It has generally been doubted that active specific immunotherapy (ASI) can be successful in inducing regressions in human metastatic disease [5]; indeed, many attempts using tumor cell-derived preparations extensively tested in the tumor-bearing patients during the 1970s and early 1980s were ineffective [6] and have largely been abandoned. However, several investigators do assert that ASI can be an effective modality in minimal residual tumor cell burdens [8, 29] and accumulating clinical evidence suggests that appropriate immunization procedures can be used to generate clinically meaningful ASI, especially against renal cell carcinoma (RCC) [14, 15, 28, 30].

The adjuvants with unspecific stimulatory activity utilized in these clinical studies included bacillus Calmette-Guérin [7, 30], *Corynebacterium parvum* [15, 27, 28], and Newcastle disease virus (NDV) [24]. Animal studies showed some evidence for the antitumor activity of the agents in vivo [8, 9, 29]. It is desirable to improve the therapeutic effect of the cancer vaccines presenting presumably weakly immunogenic relevant antigens by selecting more suitable adjuvants. In a previous study we demonstrated that recombinant interleukin-2 (rIL-2) can serve an effective adjuvant function when administered with an RCC vaccine in patients after nephrectomy without remaining macroscopic evidence of the disease [24].

In the patients immunized *with the addition of IL-2*, an augmentation of delayed-type hypersensitivity (DTH) response to ASI including an increasing reaction to unmodified autologous tumor cells

[1] Chirurgische Universitätsklinik, Abteilung Urologie, Im Neuenheimer Feld 110, W-6900 Heidelberg, FRG
[2] Deutsches Krebsforschungszentrum, Institut für Immunologie und Genetik, Im Neuenheimer Feld 280, W-6900 Heidelberg, FRG

G. Staehler S. Pomer (Eds.)
Basic and Clinical Research on Renal Cell Carcinoma

was documented. Patients vaccinated with NDV-modified autologous tumor cells *without IL-2* showed no increase in the DTH reactivity throughout repeated vaccinations.

IL-2 has been used in therapy for RCC in many preclinical and clinical studies [26, 32]. Following the clinical demonstration of augmented antitumor activity of IL-2 in RCC by combining it with recombinant interferon-alpha (IFN-α) using either high-dose bolus intravenous therapy [26] or long-term subcutaneous administration [1] we used rIL-2/rIFN-α-2b therapy with the latter approach in combination with ASI.

This is a report of our experience with sequential vaccination with autologous NDV-modified tumor cells using (rIL-2) as a local adjuvant for the coinjection with tumor cells and low-dose subcutaneous administation of rIL-2 and rIFN-α in patients with metastatic RCC.

Material and Methods

Patient Population

Thirty patients with advanced RCC were treated by vaccination with NDV-modified autologous tumor cells combined with low-dose rIL-2 and IFN-α-2b. Of these, 23 patients suffered from metastasizing cancer with distant lesions to at least one organ, while 7 patients were considered to be at high risk of developing early metastases because of the histologic grading (G = III), tumor size (T = 3b, 4) or vena cava invasion (V2). Local lymph node involvement was seen in seven patients. The criteria for acceptance of patients to this study were histologic verification of the primary tumor, absence of brain metastases, and recovery from the surgery. Immunotherapy was started as soon as the patients recovered from the nephrectomy, usually 3 weeks after the operation. Written informed consent was received from every patient.

Tumor Procurement, Dissociation and Cryopreservation

After resection, the kidney specimen were opened immediately under sterile conditions. All tumor tissue not required for staging and 5 g of normal kidney were excised, placed in sterile tubes with RPMI solution, and carried immediately on ice to the laboratory for processing and freezing. The tissue dissociation procedure of Kemmner et al. [13] was used under sterile conditions in a laminar flow hood. After washing twice with phosphate-buffered saline (PBS) to remove the debris and erythrocytes, the remaining tumor fragments were transferred to an Erlenmeyer flask containing the PBS solution and glass beads. The standard enzyme cocktail consisted of collagenase IV (41.6 mg/100 ml), hyaluronidase (33.0 mg/100 dl) and DNase (15.4 mg/100 dl; Sigma, Munich) dissolved in Hank's balanced salt solution (HBSS) at pH 7.2, i.e., the pH optimum of collagenase. Tissue pieces were incubated for 30 min at 37°C under gentle agitation with a magnetic stirrer. The suspension was then collected and pooled through a steel mesh, collected and centrifuged at 110 *g* for 10 min at 4 °C and resuspended in PBS. The procedure was repeated with the remaining fragments two or three times, depending on the state of the tissue. Finally, also supernatants were collected, centrifuged at 110 *g* for 10 min and then resuspended with PBS. Cell number and viability were determined by trypan blue solution. Using centrifugation through Ficoll-Hypaque (Pharmacia, Freiburg, Germany), erythrocytes and dead cells were removed.

The dissociated tumor cells were adjusted to 1.5×10^7/ml in HBSS, placed in 2-ml nunc freezer vials and transferred on ice. Before freezing 1 ml freezing medium containing 10% DMSO was added. Then controlled-rate freezing (−1 °C/min to −80 °C) was performed. The vials were transferred in liquid nitrogen to storage at −196 °C.

For the preparation of vaccine, the vial of frozen tumor cells was rapidly thawed in a 38 °C water bath, and tumor cells were diluted slowly in buffer medium, 32 Hau NDV was added and incubated in a 37°C water bath. The modified cells were placed on ice and irradiated with 20000 rad (200 Gy using a 137-Cesium source). The volume of the cell suspension was adjusted such that 10^7 viable tumor cells remained in the tubes. The vaccine suspensions were drawn into a 1.0-ml syringe. The syringes were placed on ice for transport to the clinic ward.

Study Design: ASI and Drug Regimen

The patients were immunized intradermaly into the thigh according to a special protocol at least twice at bi-weekly intervals. Starting usually on day 21 after the operation the patients were vaccinated in a chessboard manner with different amounts of tumor cells, virus, and 75000 U rIL-2 either separately or in combination. On several occasions as well normal kidney cells were used for specificity. Then a subcutaneous regimen of rIL-2 plus rIFN-α-2b was implemented.

The rIFN-α-2b used in this study was supplied to the group by ESSEX-Schering (Munich, FRG) and rIL-2 by Eurocetus (Amsterdam, Netherlands).

Each course of treatment consisted of a 2-week cycle during which rIL-2 1.5 million cetus U/m^2 per day was given on days 1 and 2 and 0.75 million cetus U/m^2 per day was administered together with rIFN-α-2b, 3 million U/m^2 per day on days 3, 5 and 8, 10, and 12. The injections were given at 12-h intervals on an outpatient basis.

Assessment of Response. Patients' tumor status was assessed every 6 weeks (but blood counts were done weekly). Complete remission was defined as the disappearance of all clinical and laboratory signs of disease; partial remission as at least 50% reduction in the sum of the products of the greatest perpendicular diameters of measurable lesions without an increase in size of any lesion, or the appearance of new lesions; stable disease as less than a partial response in the absence of disease progression for at least 8 weeks; and disease progression as an increase of at least 25% in the sum of the products of the longest perpendicular diameters of measurable lesions, or the development of new lesions.

Results

Of 30 treated patients 23 were eligible and evaluable for response. Seven patients had no evaluable lesion after surgery of metastases and were included in a separate analysis of the adjuvant immunotherapy with ASI and subcutaneous rIL-2. In this report only toxicity was assessed. Of these 23 patients 20 received at least 3 cycles (6 weeks) of therapy. The treatment was tolerated quite well. There was no severe toxicity (WHO grade 3 and 4). None of the patients required transfusion for anemia or treatment for capillary leak-induced swelling and weight gain, fluid retention or hypovolemia. Side effects such as fever, malaise, nausea, diarrhea, focal inflammation at the injection site always resolved after cessation of the therapy.

Nonresponders. In one patient progression of bone metastases was very rapid. Despite complete disappearance of several lung metastases within 2 weeks (one cycle) of the start of the treatment, the performance status of the patient deteriorated due to hastened progression of bone disease and the therapy was discontinued during the third course. There were two other discontinuations of the treatment regimen in the third cycle: in one patient a brain metastasis was detected; in another patient with progressing disease the dose was escalated and a 5-day continuous infusion started with no subsequent remission seen. There were three deaths thus far in the patients mentioned with progressing disease.

In six of nine nonresponders early, slow, substantial disease progression was seen, i.e., the development of new tumor lesions or an over 25% increase in measurable lesions within 6 months. All six consented to be kept on treatment during additional treatment courses.

In the other three nonresponders intravenous dose escalation was attempted, but only 1 succeeded in reaching an individual maximal tolerated dose of 30×10^6 cetus U/m^2 per week for 4 weeks. The other two with a poorer performance status have not tolerated the high-dose i.v. treatment schedule for more than 5 and 10 days, respectively. No objective antitumor responses were noted in these patients.

Responders. Therapeutic activity was considerable. Three patients had complete remissions with disappearance of several lung metastases, and four patients had partial remissions with more than 50% regression of lung and liver metastases, respectively.

Seven patients showed stable disease during treatment courses, which were given intermittently. Since tumor regressions after IL-2 may be seen late, they were kept on treatment either until progression occurred (in three) or until they withdrew their consent (in four).

Discussion

Choice of ASI Regimen

Several specific forms of immunotherapy had already been tried in the renal cancer [14, 20, 28, 30]. The rationale was to combine within the vaccine an adjuvant with a specific component, i.e., tumor cells expressing a tumor-associated antigen, of whatever nature, thereby including and activating the host's possibly tumor specific T-cell mediated immune system [29]. Our clinical protocol was born out of the investigations with NDV-modified autologous tumor cells within the ESb tumor model system [9] and clinical experience with ASI for human colorected cancer [11, 12], malignant melanoma [4], and lung cancer [10]. Common to all these protocols was the use of autologous, highly viable tumor cells not damaged by dissociation and cryopreservation procedures. Our interest in NDV for modification of tumor cells to increase immunogenicity was due to its potency to induce interferon [3] and its low pathogenicity in humans [29].

The uniformly increased DTH reactivity to autologous tumor cells seen in our patients following the immunization confirms the sustained antigenic stimulus of the vaccine to the regional lymph nodes. It is the concomitant administration of low-dose IL-2 which causes the increased skin reactivity to the autologous tumor material [24]. The specifity, type, and inducers of cells involved in this response are under examination.

Mechanism of Action

Analyzing the mechanism of the responsiveness to the combined ASI and subcutaneous rIL-2/rIFN-α-2b therapy we cannot rule out the possibility that assuming a specific T-cell response can be elicited upon immunization of patients with inactivated autologous tumor cells, rIL-2 acts by *augmenting* the specific responses against the tumor cell vaccine. The role of IL-2 as a vaccine adjuvant in humans has just recently come under investigation [21, 31]. IL-2 has been effective with a hepatitis-B vaccine, when injected at the site of vaccination for generating protective antibody titers in chronic dialysis patients unresponsive to previous immunization attempts [17]. IL-2 boosted the immune response and antibody titers against the hepatitis-B membrane antigen in seven of ten patients, whereas in the control group receiving the vaccine along just one of eight patients developed protective antibody titers.

The effectiveness of lymphokines in generating responses to human *tumor cell* vaccines is currently under intensive scrutiny. Knowing that multilymphokine supernatants boost responses to tumor cell vaccines [22], McCune and Marquis [16] have studied the potential of IL-1 to serve as an adjuvant in a murine tumor model when administered either locally with the vaccine or given systemically.

IL-1 was highly effective in its adjuvant function. Even when IL-1 was injected at a remote site from the vaccine, it functioned as well as when given at the vaccine site, indicating that this lymphokine acts as a systemic adjuvant. The possibility of the antitumor action resulting from cytotoxic effects of IL-1 was excluded by the experimental design; the IL-1 was given at least 7 days before the tumor challenge was started.

The mechanisms of unresponsiveness to hepatitis-B vaccine in chronic dialysis patients and to tumor cell vaccines in the cancer patients are different and result from immunosuppression and from poor antigenicity, respectively.

But a common element of both the therapy concepts was stimulating the production of specifically sensitized lymphocytes. As the first step ASI activated in vivo specific T cells against autologous residual tumor. This was followed by expansion of the population of tumor-sensitized T cells by IL-2 therapy.

Our schedule of treatment was not associated with significant toxicity. We preferred not to exclude older patients with marginal performance, especially with marginal cardiac or pulmonary status, from the study. These patients interrupted treatment for 2 to 3-week periods of rest. Clinical experience has suggested that long, tolerable, "steady disease" periods with no dramatic, measurable response and no sign of progression were achieved in these patients.

It appears that the sequential administration of ASI and subcutaneous low-dose rIL-2/rIFN-α-2b in this schedule is feasible and effective. The overall response rate of 33% is similar to the results obtained with the high-toxicity intravenous IL-2 regimens [19, 26, 32], long-term subcutaneous administration of rIL-2 and rIFN-α-2b [1], most effective combination of tumor necrosis factor (TNF) and rIFN-α-2b [23] and the biologically active dosage of recombinant IFN-γ [2].

We conclude that sequential therapy using an autologous, cryopreserved irradiated tumor cell vaccine followed by outpatient therapy with recombinant IL-2/interferon-α administered subcutaneously shows significant salutary effects, is a remarkable safe, and low in toxicity. We currently are conducting randomized trial in patients with metastasizing RCC (ASI + IL-2/IFN-α-2b vs IL-2/IFN-α-2b without ASI) to assess the role of ASI within the combined treatment regimen.

References

1. Atzpodien J, Körfer A, Franks CR, Poliwoda H, Kirchner H (1990) Home therapy with recombinant interleukin-2 andinterferon-α-2b in advanced human malignancies. Lancet 335: 1509–1512

2. Aulitzky W, Gastl G, Aulitzki WE, Herold M, Kemmler J, Mull B, Frick J, Huber Ch (1989) Successful treatment of metastatic renal cell carcinoma with a biologically active dose of recombinant Interferon-gamma. J Clin Oncol 7/12: 1875–1884
3. Brown CL, Peters PC, Prager MD, Baechtel S (1981) Specific immunotherapy of metastatic renal cell carcinoma. Proc of AUA, Boston, Abstr 337
4. Cassel WA, Murray DR, Phillips H (1983) A phase II study on the postsurgical management of stage II malignant melanoma with a Newcastle Disease Virus Oncolysate. Cancer 52: 856–860
5. Fauci AS (1987) Immunomodulators in clinical medicine. Ann Intern Med 106: 421–433
6. Fowler JE (1986) Failure of immunotherapy for metastatic renal cell carcinoma. J Urol 135: 22
7. Galligioni E, Francini M, Carbone A, et al. (1989) Specific delayed type cutaneous hypersensitivity (DTCH) to autolougs tumor in renal cancer patients treated with active specific immunotherapy (ASI). Proc ASCO 8: Abstr 690, p 178
8. Hanna MG, Hoover HC, Peters LC, et al. (1987) Fundamental and applied aspects of successful active specific immunotherapy of cancer. In: Oldham R (ed) Cancer biotherapy principles and practice. Raven Press, New York, pp 195–221
9. Heicappell R, Schirrmacher V, von Hoegen P, Ahlert T, Appelhans B (1986) Prevention of metastatic spread by postoperative immunotherapy with virally modified autologous tumor cells. I. Parameters for optimal therapeutic effects. Int J Cancer 37: 569–577
10. Hollinshead A, Stewart THM, Takita H, Dalvow M, Concannon J (1987) Adjuvant specific active lung cancer immunotherapy trials Tumor-associated antigens. Cancer 60: 1249–1262
11. Hoover HC, Surdyke MG, Dangel RB (1985) Prospectively randomized trial of adjuvant active specific immunotherapy for human colorectal cancer. Cancer 55: 1236–1243
12. Hoover HC, Surdyke MG, Brandhorst JS (1990) Five-year follow-up of a controlled trial of active specific immunotherapy in colorectal cancer. Proc Am Soc Clin Oncol 9: 106
13. Kemmner W, Schlag P, Brossmer R (1987) A rapid and simple procedure for dissociation of tumour tissue from the human colon. J Cancer Res Clin Oncol 113: 400–401
14. Kurth KH, Marguet R, Zwartendij KJ, Warmaar SO (1987) Autologous anticancer antigen reparation for specific immunotherapy in advanced renal cell carcinoma. Eur Urol 13: 103–109
15. McCune CS, Schapira DV, Henshaw EC (1981) Specific immunotherapy of advanced renal carcinoma: evidence for the polyclonality of metastases. Cancer 47: 1984–1987
16. McCune CS, Marquis DM (1990) Interleukin 1 as an adjuvant for active specific immunotherapy in a murine tumor model. Cancer Res 50: 1212–1215
17. Meuer SC, Dumann H, Buschenfelde KM, et al. (1989) Low-dose interleukin-2 induces systemic immune responses against HBsAg in immunodeficient non-responders to hepatitis B vaccination. Lancet 1: 15–17

18. Mitchell MS, Kempf RA, Harel W, et al. (1988) Effectiveness and tolerability of low-dose cyclophosphamide and low-dose intravenous interleukin-2 in disseminated malignant melanoma. J Clin Oncol 6: 409–424
19. Negrier S, Philip T, Stoter G, et al. (1989) Interleukin-2 with or without LAK cells in metastatic renal cell carcinoma: a report of a European multicentre study. Eur J Cancer Clin Oncol 25: 21–28
20. Neidhardt JA, Murphy SG, Hennick LA, Wise HA (1980) Active specific immunotherapy of stage for renal carcinoma with aggregated tumour antigen adjuvant. Cancer 46: 1128–1134
21. Numberg JH, Doyled MV, York SM, et al. (1989) Interleukin 2 acts as an adjuvant to increase the potency of inactivated rabies virus vaccine. Proc Natl Acad Sci USA 86: 4240–4243
22. O'Donnell RW, Marquis RW, Mudholkar GS, McCune CS (1986) In vivo enhancement of antitumor immunity by interleukin 2-rich lymphokines. Cancer Res 46: 3273–3278
23. Otto U, Schneider AW, Conrad S, Klosterhalfen H (1990) Combined therapy with TNF- und -2a Interferon. J Urol 143: 292A
24. Pomer S, Thiele R, Staehler G (1989) Die Behandlung des fortgeschrittenen Nierenzellkarzinoms mittels kombinierter Vakzinierung mit modifiziertem autologem Tumormaterial und Interleukin-2. Methodencharakterisierung und vorläufige Ergebnisse. In: Hofstetter A, Staehler G, Kriegmair M, Schuth J (eds) Zytokine in der urologischen Onkologie. Aktuelle Onkologie, vol 57. Zuckschwerdt, München, pp 28–37
25. Pomer S, Thiele R, Schirrmacher V, Staehler G (1989) Augmentation of DTH reactivity to active specific immunotherapy by local application of IL-2 in patients with renal cell carcinoma. Nat Immun Cell Growth Regul 9: 66
26. Rosenberg SA, Lotze MT, Muul LM, et al. (1987) A progress report on the treatment of 157 patients with advanced cancer using lymphokine-activated killer cells and interleukin-2 or high-dose interleukin-2 alone. N Engl J Med 316: 880–897
27. Sahasrabudhe DM, deKernion JB, Pontes JE, et al. (1986) Specific immunotherapy with suppressor function inhibition in metastatic renal cell carcinoma. J Biol Resp Mod 5: 581–594
28. Schärfe T, Becht E, Klippel KF, Jacobi GH, Hohenfellner R (1986) Active immunotherapy of stage IV renal cell cancer using autologous tumor cells. World J Urol 3: 245–248
29. Schirrmacher V, Heicappell R (1987) Prevention of metastatic spread by postoperative immunotherapy with virally modified autologous tumor cells. II. Establishment of specific systemic anti tumor immunity. Clin Exp Metastasis 5: 147–156
30. Tallberg T, Tykkä H (1986) Specific active immunotherapy in advanced renal cell carcinoma. A clinical longterm follow-up study. World J Urol 3: 234–244
31. Weinberg A, Merigan TC (1988) Recombinant interleukin 2 as an adjuvant for vaccine-induced protection. J Immunol 140: 294–299
32. West WH, Tauer KW, Yannelli JR (1987) Constant infusion recombinant interleukin-2 in adoptive immunotherapy of advanced cancer. N Engl J Med 316: 898–905

Interleukin-2 by Inhalation: Local Therapy for Metastatic Renal Cell Carcinoma

E. Huland[1], H. Huland[1], and H. Heinzer[1]

Introduction

Continuous high-dose local administration of natural interleukin-2 (nIL-2) is tolerated without side effects in advanced-cancer patients and induces complete remission and local and systemic immunoactivation, as we have shown previously [8]. Those facts support our belief that interleukins should be administered locally, rather than systemically, for effective treatment of carcinoma. Local administration can be expected to induce fewer side effects and to activate tumor-infiltrating immune cells, which are reported to be 100 times more cytotoxic than activated blood cells [11]. The local use of interleukins is also more economical in that it reduces renal loss of small molecules. Although metastatic tumor disease seems not to be suitable for a local approach, the addition of local immunoactivation to systemic treatment might improve the therapeutic effectiveness without increasing toxicity.

Of patients with metastatic renal cell carcinoma, 60%–80% have pulmonary metastases. The surface of the lung measures about 100 m^2 and thus constitutes a huge area for reaching local immune cells [3]. We present the toxicity, efficacy, and duration of therapy to response in six patients treated with long-term inhalation IL-2 combined with low-dose intravenous IL-2 and subcutaneous interferon-α.

[1] Klinikum Steglitz der Freien Universität, Urologische Klinik, Hindenburgdamm 30, W-1000 Berlin 45, FRG

G. Staehler S. Pomer (Eds.)
Basic and Clinical Research on Renal Cell Carcinoma

Materials and Methods

Patient Characteristics

Characteristics of the patients are summarized in Table 1. All patients had histologically confirmed renal cell carcinoma. Informed consent was given by each patient before entry. Patients with clinically significant cardiac disease, active infection requiring systemic antibiotic therapy, or central nervous system metastases were excluded from the study. The study was approved by the institutional review board of the Klinikum Steglitz, Free University of Berlin, Berlin, FRG.

Products

Natural human IL-2 was obtained from Biotest Pharma GmbH, Frankfurt/M., FRG. It was produced from phorbolmyristateacetate- and calciumionophor A23187-stimulated, pooled, freshly donated human mononuclear cells. The product, highly purified and free of lectins and endotoxins, was tested for the absence of several lymphokine activities: IL-1, IL-3, interferon-α, macrophage-activating factor, leukocyte migration-inhibiting factor, glucocorticoid-inducing factor,

Table 1. Characteristics of the six patients, (mean age, 54 years; range, 47–61 years)

	No. of patients
Male/female	4/2
ECOG score:	
0	2
1	1
2	2
3	1
Weight loss in previous 6 months	2
Time from initial diagnosis:	
more than 1 year	3
less than 1 year	3
Prior therapy:	
Nephrectomy	6
Interferon α_{2b}	4
Hormones	1
Radiation	1
Chemotherapy	1
Operation at metastatic site	1

macrophage migration-inhibiting factor, granulocyte-macrophage colony-stimulating factor, tumor necrosis factor α, lymphotoxin, mitogenic factor, and granulocyte chemiluminescence-activating factor. The specific activity of nIL-2 was 10^7 U/mg of protein; the units were biological response modifier program (BRMP) units.

The nIL-2 was supplied as a solution containing 100000 U/ml in 0.01 *M* phosphate buffer with 0.15 *M* NaCl at a pH of 7.4 and with 0.1% (v/v) human serum albumin; it was used for inhalation without further dilution.

Recombinant interferon-α_{2b} was purchased from Essex/Schering, Munich, FRG.

Natural human interferon-α was supplied by the German Red Cross as a solution with a specific activity of $4–5 \times 10^7$ U/mg of protein. The concentration of solution was 3×10^6 U/ml.

Treatment

The treatment schedule is shown in Fig. 1.

Natural IL-2 inhalation of 100000 U nIL-2 was performed with a Salvia Lifetec nebulizer five times per day continuously throughout the study.

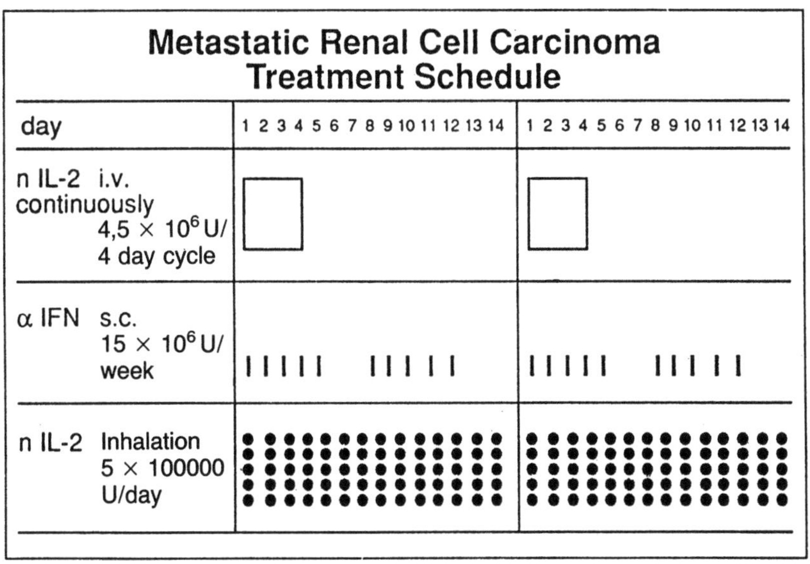

Fig. 1. Treatment schedule

Every 2 weeks, a 4-day cycle of intravenous nIL-2 was administered – a total dose of 4.5 million U dissolved in 500 ml of phosphate buffer with 0.5% human serum albumin was given continuously. If it was well tolerated, the dose of nIL-2 was increased.

Recombinant Interferon-α_{2b} and Natural Interferon-α. Patients were given 3×10^6 U subcutaneously once a day 5 days/week, usually in the evening. Four patients were treated with recombinant interferon-α and two patients with natural interferon-α.

Medication During Therapy. During intravenous administration of nIL-2, four doses of 0.5 g of paracetamol were given to patients routinely. Aspisol was given intravenously if body temperature exceeded 39 °C. During inhalation therapy alone, no medication was necessary. Subcutaneous administration of interferon-α in some patients required anti-inflammatory medication because of fever. Paracetamol and aspirin were prescribed.

Blood

Complete urinary analysis and blood analysis for the following characteristics were carried out before treatment, at least three times during each intravenous cycle, and once a week during inhalation therapy: complete blood-cell count, platelet count, serum electrolytes, creatinine, bilirubin, albumin, serum glutamic-oxaloacetictransaminase (SGOT), serum glutamic-pyruvic transaminase (SGPT), calcium, and magnesium.

Toxicity

Each patient had an ECG before treatment and before each intravenous cycle. Patients were hospitalized during intravenous cycles. Transfer to the intensive care unit was not necessary. Toxicity was graded according to WHO criteria.

Measurement of Response

Each patient underwent physical examination and a chest X-ray before treatment and every 2 weeks during therapy and bone scanning and computed tomographic (CT) scanning of lungs, abdomen and pelvis before treatment and every 3 months thereafter.

Response criteria were as follows: A reduction of at least 50% in the sum of the products of the perpendicular diameters of all measurable lesions constituted a partial response. A reduction of less than 50% constituted stable disease. An increase of at least 25% constituted progressive disease. ECOG scores were obtained every 4 weeks. Mean survival was compared with estimated survival according to risk criteria [5].

Results

Immunotherapy

The mean duration of therapy is 183 days (range, 97–296), and treatment continues in all patients.

Patient 1, with lung metastasis only, refused intravenous nIL-2 after 12 cycles, but continued successfully with inhalation nIL-2 and subcutaneous interferon-α for another 4 months, with continuous reduction of pulmonary metastases (Fig. 2a, b).

The median intravenous dose per cycle was 4.6 million U. An increase in the intravenous dose was tolerated better during earlier cycles than during the later ones.

Five times per day, patients inhaled 100000 U of nIL-2 on an ambulatory basis without problems. An increase to 300000 U five times per day was tolerated extremely well, but patients complained that therapy became too time-consuming.

Tumor Response

All six patients could be evaluated (Table 2). Responses correlated directly with sites of metastasis.

Lung. Five patients had lung metastases including two who had no other metastases. All lung metastases responded to therapy (Figs. 2–4).

Pleura. One patient had a single pleural metastasis with diffuse pulmonary metastases. Despite partial pulmonary response, the pleural metastasis progressed; surgical removal of this metastasis is planned.

Table 2. Response to treatment

Site of metastatic disease	No. of patients	Response[a]	Duration of response (months, since response began)
Lung	5	PR[b]	9+, 9+, 5+ 3+, 2+
Lung only	2	PR[b]	9+, 3+,
Pleura	1	PD	
Mediastinum	2	SD	
Liver	1	SD	
Abdomen and Pelvis	2	SD	
Bone	3	PD	

[a] *PR*, partial response; *SD*, stable disease; *PD*, progressive disease
[b] with continuing regression of tumor

Mediastinum, Liver, Abdomen, and Pelvis. Four patients had soft-tissue metastases at these sites. All remained stable. The observation time was 4, 5, 5, and 10 months.

Bone. Three patients had bone metastases. All progressed during therapy. Surgical resection in two patients was performed after 3 months of therapy because of bone instability and one had a surgical resection after 9 months.

Development of New Metastases. Despite long periods of observation of some patients, no new metastases were diagnosed at any site during therapy.

ECOG Score

The two patients with the most unfavorable ECOG score improved through successful tumor treatment. Patient 1 had an ECOG performance status of 3 on entry into the study. He suffered from severe respiratory distress, caused by disseminated pulmonary metastases, at the slightest activity (Fig. 2). He had previously lost 24 kg of weight (from 80 to 56 kg). His symptoms abated considerably after 4 weeks of therapy; he gained 15 kg of weight and his ECOG performance status is now 1.

Patient 3 had an ECOG performance status of 2, which is now 1. Besides distinct tumor reduction in the lung, successful operation

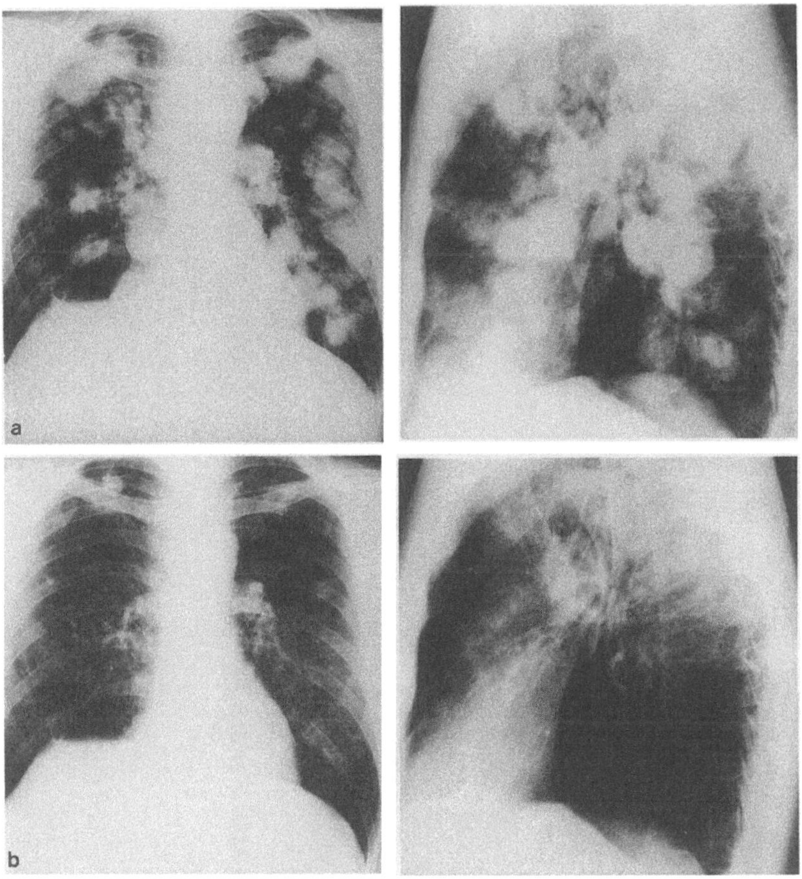

Fig. 2. **a** Chest X-ray of patient 1 before treatment (12/89). **b** Chest X-ray of patient 1 after 9 months of treatment (9/90)

for a painful vertebral metastasis has improved the quality of this patient's life.

Four patients remained stable. Three of them had satisfactory ECOG scores (1 and 0). The fourth, who is stable with an ECOG performance status of 2, has no lung metastases and stable liver metastases.

Survival

The first three patients who entered the study can be evaluated as having exceeded their median survival, which by risk-assessment

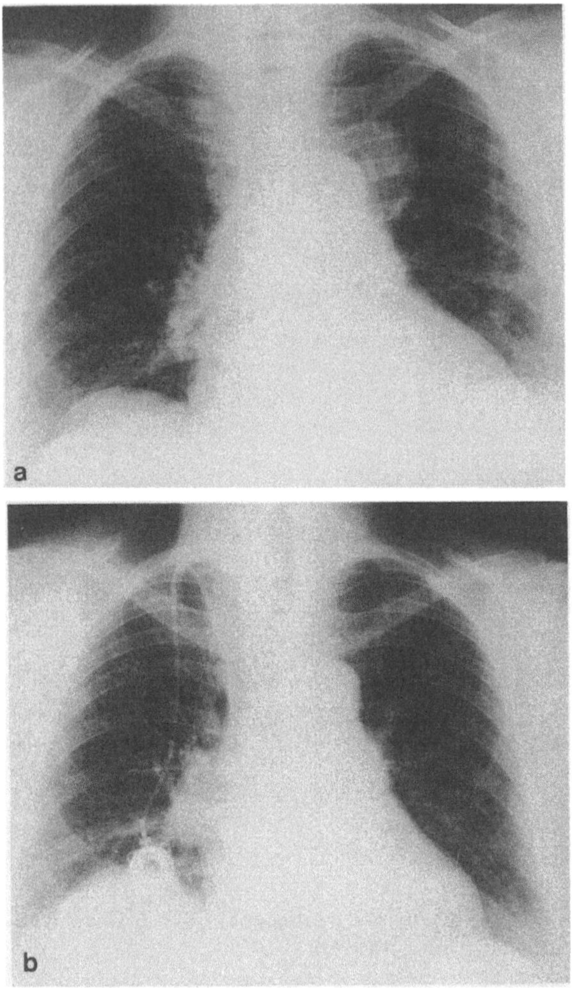

Fig. 3. **a** Chest X-ray of patient 3 before treatment (5/90). **b** Chest X-ray of patient 3 after 4 months of treatment (9/90)

criteria [5] had been estimated at 2.1, 5.3, and 5.3 months. Follow-up times of these patients are now 10, 10, and 6 months, respectively.

Toxicity

Patients' Assessment. According to the patients, intravenous nIL-2 treatment impaired their performance status mostly. Interferon-α

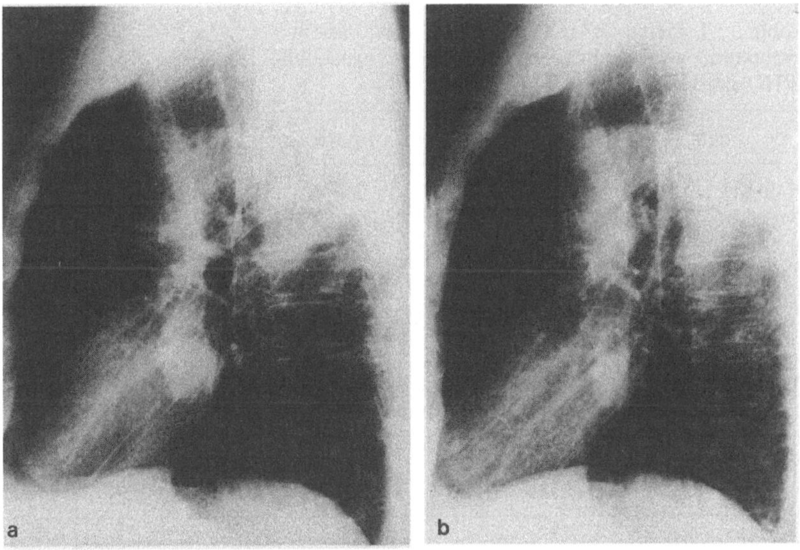

Fig. 4. **a** Chest X-ray of patient 5 before treatment (7/90). **b** Chest X-ray of patient 5 after 2 months of treatment (9/90)

given on an ambulatory basis by 4 of 6 patients was judged clearly to impair their lives. However, it was considered less impairing than intravenous nIL-2. Inhaled nIL-2 was tolerated extremely well. The patients reported that nausea was best suppressed by eating before inhalation. Patients considered transient morning cough as mild. Some patients complained about the duration of inhalation – about 15–30 min per administration (Table 3).

Objective Assessment. Inhaled nIL-2 produced no toxic effects in blood. Other toxic side effects were considered mild (Table 3). Inhalation treatment was administered on an outpatient basis.

Sixty cycles of intravenous nIL-2 were evaluated for adverse effects. Toxicity was moderate, not exceeding WHO grade 1, except for fever, hypotension and nausea, which were classified in many cycles as grade 2 (Table 4). Bilirubin, SGOT, and SGPT remained normal during all cycles. Transient increase in serum alkaline phosphatase occurred in nine cycles in two patients. Capillary leak-induced fluid retention and weight gain did not occur. No patient needed transfusion for thrombocytopenia or anemia. No adverse effects on the central nervous system were observed.

Table 3. Toxicity of inhaled nIL-2 (six patients evaluated; all effects were mild; none exceeded WHO grade 1)

Side effects	No. of patients
Nausea	3
Dry skin	2
Arthralgia	4
Fatigue	6
Cough	3

Table 4. Toxicity of combined intravenous nIL-2, inhaled nIL-2 and subcutaneous interferon-α (60 cycles evaluated)

Side effect	No. of cycles		
	WHO Grade 0	WHO Grade 1	WHO Grade 2
Fever	0	9	51
Hypotension	0	3	57
Nausea and vomiting	0	48	12
Malaise	0	60	0
Diarrhea	51	9	0
Anorexia	23	37	0
Skin reactivity	38	22	0
Respiratory distress	48	12	0
Renal insufficiency	38	22	0
Liver toxicity	60	0	0
Arrhythmia	60	0	0
Peripheral polyneuropathy	56	4	0
Arthralgia	53	7	0
Alopecia	44	16	0
Infection	58	0	2
Edema	60	0	0
Fatigue	11	49	0

Hematologic Effects

Peripheral blood eosinophils – according to previous results not considered to be toxic [7] – increased overall from 177/μl before therapy to 1163/μl during inhalation therapy ($p < 0.05$) and to 3418/μl during additional intravenous cycles ($p < 0.05$). There was no statistical difference between absolute eosinophil count in inhalation only and in additional intravenous IL-2 therapy.

Operative Treatment During Immunotherapy

Three patients had bone metastases, all of which progressed during therapy. Two of those underwent surgery because of danger of instability after 3 months of treatment. One of those was operated on for a slow-growing pelvic metastasis. No other bone metastasis has developed in any patients so far.

Infection During Therapy

After 4 weeks of inhalation, patient 1 developed pneumonia. Because tumor response was good, inhalation treatment was continued, and pneumonia was treated successfully with intravenous administration of antibiotics for 2 weeks. One patient had an infection of an implanted catheter system, which was treated successfully with administration of antibiotics and removal of the catheter.

Discussion

This first report of administration of IL-2 by inhalation demonstrates extremely low toxicity and provides a schedule for long-term ambulatory application. The latter is important because long-term treatment seems to be essential for continued antitumor response: distinct pulmonary responses were observed after 4 weeks of therapy, but further reduction of pulmonary metastases required long-term treatment. Moreover, a low-toxicity schedule can now be offered to patients in poor condition.

This new type of interleukin administration achieved a response rate not described before [13, 9, 2, 1]. Response was directly correlated with metastatic site. Distinct tumor reduction was achieved in almost all lung metastases, even without additional intravenous nIL-2 administration. No pulmonary metastasis grew during inhalation treatment.

The influence of additional systemic interleukins on response rates in our protocol requires further evaluation. However, comparable response rates in the lung cannot be achieved by exclusively systemic therapy with comparable or even higher doses of intravenous nIL-2 [12, 14, 10]. Treatment success also cannot be ascribed only to interferon-α, inasmuch as four patients had been pretreated with interferon-α as a single cytokine without success.

Local nIL-2 administration in patients with advanced tumor induces a systemic increase in IL-2 receptor-positive cells, as we have shown previously [8]. IL-2 receptor-positive cells are likely to originate from the IL-2-treated tumor and may develop not only systemic antitumor activity but may also transport immunological information and induce systemic immune responses. This should be a subject of further studies. Systemic IL-2 was added in our protocol to support locally activated immune cells re-entering the circulation. In addition to the clear benefit for patients with lung metastases, patients with metastases at other sites might benefit. Activation of immune cells in the lung might enhance a systemic immune response without increasing toxicity. Except for bone metastases and the single pleural metastasis, nonpulmonary metastases stabilized in our patients, and new metastases did not develop during therapy. These results could be clinical correlates of concomitant immunity, an experimentally induced phenomenon in animals in which a host bearing a progressive tumor can destroy a small implant of cells of the tumor given at distant sites [6]. In animal experiments, concomitant tumor immunity has functioned as an important defense mechanism against tumor metastasis [4]. Effective prevention of new metastases could give rise to a broader spectrum of operative indications for treating single or not completely responding metastases or for shortening treatment time with cytokines. In our study, three patients had additional bone metastases; all were operated on successfully.

We learned from our pilot study that decrease in pulmonary lesions continues even after 10 months of treatment – a strong argument for long-term, or even lifelong, therapy, although this needs to be confirmed in further studies. However, this pilot study showed that long-term IL-2 inhalation treatment is possible because of its extremely low toxicity.

None of the six patients has died after a mean follow-up of 183 days (range 97–296 days). Although none of the patients had a complete response, survival clearly was prolonged. Two patients in poor condition had significant improvements in ECOG score and body weight. Despite the continuation of treatment, the quality of patients' lives had improved considerably, and both are back at work.

Vascular leakage or pulmonary edema did not occur in any of the patients. It might be important whether IL-2 induces the cytokine cascade from tissue site or from endothelial site. A distinct increase in eosinophil leukocytes during treatment was seen in all patients. As we have shown previously [7, 8], there is evidence that eosinophil leukocytes are involved in the antitumor response and do not have to be considered as indications of toxicity. Natural human IL-2 was used for inhalation therapy because of its stability and solubility without additives. In light of our data, it cannot necessarily be concluded that recombinant *E. coli*-derived nonglycosylated IL-2 is as effective and nontoxic in inhalation therapy. In particular, it might not be desirable to inhale additives (e.g., SDS), which could be toxic.

Despite the small number of patients, the clinical results of our study have important implications for further studies and encourage us to pursue the principle of local administration of interleukins in these and other tumors.

References

1. Atzpodien J, Körfer A, Franks CR, et al. (1990) Home therapy with recombinant interleukin-2 and interferon-α2b in advanced human malignancies. Lancet 335: 1509
2. Bergmann L, Weidmann E, Mitrou PS, et al. (1990) Interleukin-2 in combination with interferon-alpha in disseminated malignant melanoma and advanced renal cell carcinoma. A phase I/II study. Onkologie 13: 137
3. Daniele RP (ed) (1988) Immunology and immunologic diseases of the lung. Blackwell Scientific Publ, Oxford
4. Dye ES (1986) The antimetastatic function of concomitant antitumor immunity. J Immunol 136: 1510
5. Elson PJ, Witte RS, Trump DL (1988) Prognostic factors for survival in patients with recurrent or metastatic renal cell carcinoma. Cancer Res 48: 7310
6. Gorrelick E (1983) Concomitant tumor immunity and the resistance to a second tumor challenge. Adv Cancer Res 39: 71
7. Heinzer H, Huland E, Huland H (1990) Activated eosinophil leukocytes in interleukin-2 (IL-2) treated patients: Evidence for a new antitumor effector mechanism. J Cancer Res Clin Oncol 116 (Suppl I): 369
8. Huland E, Huland H (1989) Local continuous high dose interleukin-2: a new therapeutic model for the treatment of advanced bladder carcinoma. Cancer Res 49: 5469
9. Lee KH, Talpaz M, Rothberg JM, et al. (1989) Concomitant administration of recombinant human interleukin-2 and recombinant interferonα-2A in cancer patients: a phase I study. J Clin Oncol 7: 1726
10. Negrier S, Philip T, Stoter G, et al. (1989) Interleukin-2 with or without LAK cells in metastatic renal cell carcinoma: a report of a European multicentre study. Eur J Cancer Clin Oncol 25: 21
11. Rosenberg SA, Speiss P, Lafreniere R (1986) A new approach to the adoptive immunotherapy of cancer with tumor infiltrating lymphocytes. Science 233: 1318
12. Rosenberg SA, Lotze MT, Muul LM, et al. (1987) A progress report on the treatment of 157 patients with advanced cancer using lymphokine-activated killer cells and interleukin-2 or high-dose interleukin-2 alone. N Engl J Med 316: 880

13. Rosenberg SA, Lotze MT, Yang JC, et al. (1989) Combination therapy with interleukin-2 and alpha-interferon for the treatment of patients with advanced cancer. J Clin Oncol 7: 1863
14. West WH, Tauer KW, Yannelli JR, et al. (1987) Constant infusion-recombinant interleukin-2 in adoptive immunotherapy of advanced cancer. N Engl J Med 316: 898

Subject Index

MIX
Papier aus verantwortungsvollen Quellen
Paper from responsible sources
FSC® C105338

If you have any concerns about our products,
you can contact us on
ProductSafety@springernature.com

In case Publisher is established outside the EU,
the EU authorized representative is:
Springer Nature Customer Service Center GmbH
Europaplatz 3, 69115 Heidelberg, Germany

Printed by Libri Plureos GmbH
in Hamburg, Germany